MW00737846

Healthcare Privacy & Confidentiality

THE COMPLETE LEGAL GUIDE

Jonathan P. Tomes, J.D.

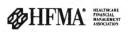

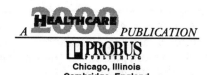

A HEALTHCARE 2000 PUBLICATION

PROBUS
PUBLISHING

Chicago, Illinois
Cambridge, England

A **2000** *HEALTHCARE PUBLICATION*

ISBN 1-55738-611-0

Printed in the United States of America

BB

1 2 3 4 5 6 7 8 9 0

BH

For Paul

Table of Contents

1

The Right to Privacy

Introduction

The Clinton administration's healthcare proposals have dramatically heightened the public's interest in the privacy and confidentiality of medical information. Visions of the personal details of their medical conditions and treatments being accessible to a computer hacker who accesses computerized patient records or electronically submitted medical claims are the basis for some of the strongest objections to the administration's plan, which calls for automating healthcare recordkeeping and claims. And the stigma and discrimination that can result from one's identification as being HIV positive or as the carrier of another sexually transmitted disease have contributed to the public's concern.

Although these concerns are certainly legitimate, so is the need for healthcare professionals to have access to private matters in order to properly treat their patients and to communicate that information with other professionals for proper purposes. An understanding of patients' rights to privacy and confidentiality in healthcare will help them treat patients properly and avoid liability for an invasion of patient privacy and confidentiality. This chapter will define the right to privacy, explain where it comes from, and discuss court decisions and statutes that have interpreted and protected the right to privacy and confidentiality. Chapter 1 concludes with a discussion of the right to privacy and confidentiality in medical ethics.

The Right to Privacy

Although our society views privacy as fundamental to the concept of individual freedom, neither the law nor society itself has defined privacy precisely. Perhaps the best definition is "the right to be left alone."[1] The right to privacy—to be left alone—actually consists of three related rights: freedom from intrusion or observation in one's private affairs, the right to maintain control over personal information, and the freedom to act without outside interference.[2]

The U.S. Constitution does not contain an explicit right of privacy, although some state constitutions do. However, as long ago as 1965, the U.S. Supreme Court found a right to privacy in the "penumbras" of the Constitution. *Penumbras* are implicit rights found as necessary corollaries of explicit rights. The right to privacy comes from the right of freedom of association in the first amendment, the prohibition against quartering soldiers in one's home in time of peace without the owner's consent found in the third amendment, the right to be free from unreasonable searches and seizures in the fourth amendment, the fifth amendment's prohibition of compulsory self-incrimination, the language of the ninth amendment that states that the "enumeration in the constitution of certain rights will not be construed to deny or disparage others retained by the people," and the fourteenth amendment's concept of personal liberty and restrictions on state action.

The Supreme Court announced the right to privacy in *Griswold v. Connecticut*[3] in reversing the convictions of an official of the Planned Parenthood League of Connecticut and a physician who had aided and abetted the use of a contraceptive drug by a married couple, finding that the statute under which they were prosecuted violated the right to privacy. After specifying those guarantees in the Bill of Rights under which the right to privacy arises, as discussed above, the court added:

> We deal with a right of privacy older than the Bill of Rights—older than our political parties, older than our school system. Marriage is a coming together for better or worse, hopefully enduring, and intimate to the degree of being sacred. It is an association that promotes a way of life, not causes; a harmony in living; not political faith; a bilateral loyalty, not commercial or social projects. Yet it is an association for as noble a purpose as any involved in our prior decisions.[4]

Thus, the states could not lawfully criminalize the use of contraceptives by married persons, because decisions concerning procreation were within the private area protected by the right to privacy. In 1972, the Supreme Court answered the question whether the right to privacy extended to reproductive decisions by the unmarried. In finding that it did, the Court stated that "if the right of privacy means anything, it is the right of the individual, married or single, to be free from unwarranted government intrusion into matters so fundamentally affecting a person as a decision whether to bear a child."[5]

Perhaps the most famous court decision concerning the right to privacy is *Roe v. Wade*.[6] In it, the Supreme Court relied on the right to privacy in finding that a woman has a right to have an abortion, although the right was a qualified one. Thus, the right to privacy prohibits the state from preventing an abortion before the fetus becomes viable. After the fetus becomes viable, the state has an important and legitimate interest in potential life and may regulate or even prevent an abortion. In his concurring opinion, Justice Douglas specified those rights he believed were implicit within the right to privacy:

- The autonomous control over the development and expression of one's intellect, interests, tastes, and personality.

- Freedom of choice in the basic decisions of one's life respecting marriage, divorce, procreation, contraception, and the education and upbringing of children.

- Freedom to care for one's health and person; freedom from bodily restraint or compulsion; freedom to walk, stroll, or loaf.[7]

Roe v. Wade and other cases indicate that the right to privacy is not absolute. Under *Roe*, the state could prevent the abortion of a fetus in the third trimester and, in other cases, the Supreme Court refused to extend the right of privacy to the use of laetrile[8] or to protect those engaging in homosexual conduct.[9] And *Webster v. Reproductive Health Services*[10] modified *Roe* by upholding a statute that, among other things, required a physician to ascertain whether the fetus was viable before performing an abortion if he or she had reason to believe the mother was 20 or more weeks pregnant; prohibited the use of public employees and facilities to perform or assist abortions not necessary to save the mother's life; and prohibited the use of public funds, employees, or facilities for the purpose of encouraging or counseling a woman to have an abortion not necessary to save her life. This decision largely returned abortion regulation to the states' political processes. States may and have enacted statutes requiring third-party consent for minor patients[11] and prohibiting the use of state facilities for performing abortions.

However, *Webster* did not do away with the right to privacy recognized in *Roe v. Wade*, and the states cannot go too far in regulating abortion. For example, in *Akron v. Akron Center for Reproductive Health*,[12] the court refused to allow a state to impose a 24-hour waiting period between the decision to seek an abortion and undergoing the surgical procedure.

State courts have also contributed to the recognition of a right to privacy, primarily in the field of tort law. In 1938, the Supreme Court of North Carolina recognized that a plaintiff could recover damages for an invasion of privacy in a case in which the defendant published the plaintiff's photograph in a newspaper advertisement without permission.[13] Among tort actions for violations of one's right to privacy are:

- *Intrusion upon a person's seclusion or solitude.* Cases involving this tort include intruding into one's bedroom and unauthorized prying into private bank accounts.[14]

- *Public disclosure of private information.* This tort consists of publicizing a matter concerning one's private life that would be highly offensive to a reasonable person and not of legitimate concern to the public. Plaintiffs have brought cases under this theory for publishing X-rays of a woman's pelvic region in a newspaper,[15] for exhibiting films of a caesarean section,[16] and for identifying the plaintiff as the teenage father of an illegitimate child.[17]

- *Placing the plaintiff in an objectionable false light in the public eye.* For example, one case found the defendant liable for using a picture of an honest taxi driver to illustrate an article on cheating taxi drivers.[18]

As a result of these cases and the public's increasing interest in the right to privacy, federal and state governments have enacted laws specifying privacy and confidentiality rights. Some states even adopted constitutional provisions to protect privacy. For example, Article I, § 22 of Alaska's constitution reads, "The right of the people to privacy is recognized and shall not be infringed." Other states protect privacy by statute.

The federal government has enacted a number of statutes protecting privacy. Perhaps the most well known is the Privacy Act of 1974, which limits governmental collection, maintenance, use, and dissemination of certain personal information and provides a right to correct wrong information.[19] The Consumer Credit Protection Act[20] requires credit-reporting agencies to follow procedures to insure accuracy, confidentiality, and the proper use of credit reports. The Right to Financial Privacy Act[21] limits federal access to records of financial institutions. Many states have similar statutes.

Every state and the federal government have statutes and administrative regulations protecting patients rights to privacy. Such statutes provide for the confidentiality of medical records, provide heightened protection for particularly sensitive information—such as HIV status, mental health, and developmental disabilities, diagnosis and treatment—and alcohol and drug abuse diagnosis and treatment. Many states also provide for patient privacy in a so-called patient bill of rights. Florida Statutes § 381.026, for example, provides that each healthcare facility or provider shall observe the following standards:

- The patient's individual dignity must be respected at all times and upon all occasions.

- Every patient who is provided healthcare services retains certain rights to privacy, which must be respected without regard to the patient's economic status or source of payment for his or her care. The patient's rights to privacy must be respected to the extent consistent with providing adequate medical care to the patient and with the efficient administration of the healthcare facility or provider's office. However, this subparagraph does not preclude necessary and discreet discussion of a patient's case or examination by appropriate medical personnel.

Even if these statutes did not exist, medical ethics recognizes a patient's rights to privacy and confidentiality. The Hippocratic Oath states, in pertinent part:

What I may see or hear in the course of the treatment or even outside of the treatment in regard to the life of men, which on no account must one spread abroad, I will keep to myself holding such things shameful to be spoken about.

This ethical principle remains important today. The Principles of Medical Ethics of the American Medical Association (AMA) continues the Hippocratic Oath's tradition of confidentiality in Principle IV:

A physician shall respect the rights of patients, of colleagues, and of other health professionals, and shall safeguard patient confidences within the constraints of the law.

The AMA amplified this principle in its Confidentiality Statement, which states that "the information disclosed to a physician during the course of the relationship between physician and patient is confidential to the greatest possible degree." The statement explains that the reason for the confidentiality requirement is that the patient should feel free to fully disclose personal, private information so that the physician can effectively provide needed services.

Conclusion

Whether patients' rights to privacy are based on the federal or a state constitution, a statute, or from medical ethics, little doubt exists that healthcare providers must respect these rights. The remainder of this book will assist you in doing so by explaining the specific areas in which patients have privacy and confidentiality rights, and detailing the legal requirements in those areas, including patients' rights to privacy, the confidentiality of medical information, heightened privacy protections for certain types of sensitive information, confidentiality of medical research information, confidentiality of peer review activities, exceptions to confidentiality, and requirements for confidentiality of financial and personal information.

Endnotes

1. Samuel Warren and Louis Brandeis, *The Right to Privacy, Harvard Law Review 4* (1890), p. 193.

2. Philip Kurland, "The Private, I," *University of Chicago Magazine* 7 (Autumn 1976) p. 8. *See* Robert S. Peck, *Extending the Constitutional right to Privacy in the New Technological Age,* 12 *Hofstra Law Review* 893 (Summer 1984).

3. 381 U.S. 479 (1965).

4. *Id.* at 484.

5. *Eisenstadt v. Baird,* 405 U.S. 438, 453 (1972). See also *Carey v. Population Services International,* 431 U.S. 678 (1977).

6. 410 U.S. 113 (1973).

7. 93 S.Ct. 739, 756-758.

8. *United States v. Rutherford,* 442 U.S. 544 (1979).

9. *Bowers v. Hardwick,* 478 U.S. 186 (1986).

10. 492 U.S. 490 (1989).

11. *See Akron v. Akron Center for Reproductive Health, Inc.,* 462 U.S. 416 (1983); *Bellotti v. Baird,* 443 U.S. 622 (1979); *Planned Parenthood of Central Missouri* v. *Danforth,* 428 *.S.52 (1976); *Hodgson* v. *Minnesota,* 110 S.Ct. 2926 (1990); *Akron* v. *Akron Center for Reproductive Health, Inc.* 110 S.Ct. 2972 (1990).

12. 110 S.Ct. 2972 (1990).

13. *Flake v. Greensboro News Co.,* 212 N.C. 780, 195 S.E. 55 (1938).

14. *Byfield v. Candler,* 33 Ga. 275, 125 S.E. 905 (1924); *Zimmerman* v. *Wilson,* 81 F.2d 247 (3d Cir. 1936).

15. *Banks v. King Features Syndicate,* 30 F.Supp. 353 (S.D.N.Y 1939).

16. *Griffin v. Medical Society,* 7 Misc.2d 549, 11 N.Y.S.2d 109 (1939).

17. *Hawkins v. Metromedia,* Inc. 288 S.C. 569, 344 S.E.2d 145 (1986).

18. *Peay v. Curtis Pub. Co.,* 78 F.Supp. 305 (D.D.C. 1948).

19. 5 U.S.C. § 552.

20. 15 U.S.C.§ 1601.

21. 12 U.S.C. § 3402.

2

Patients' Rights to Personal Privacy

Introduction

Not only do patients, as citizens, have the constitutional right to privacy discussed in Chapter 1 but also they typically have specific rights to privacy found in a so-called patient bill of rights or other statutes or regulations establishing specific privacy protections for hospital or long-term care facility patients. Aside from the right to privacy concerning their medical records and medical information, patients have a right to personal privacy under these laws. Patient privacy protections typically include the right to:

- Be treated with consideration, respect, and dignity. This right is particularly applicable to medical treatment and to personal care.

- Private communications with providers, attorneys, ombudsmen, and others who are assisting patients or handling complaints for them.

- Send and receive mail unopened.

- Have access to a telephone to make and receive calls in private.

- Privacy in treatment, living arrangements, and care for personal needs. No one whose presence is not necessary for treatment or care for personal needs should be present without the patient's consent. Facility staff should recognize patients' privacy rights in their living arrangements by knocking before entering, except in emergencies.

- If married, privacy for spousal visits. If both are patients or residents in the facility, to live together unless medically contraindicated.

- Associate with and to communicate privately with persons of their choice.

- Manage their own financial affairs, unless they delegate such duties to the facility.

Of course, the facility may limit these rights when medically contraindicated or when the exercise of such rights endangers other residents or substantially limits the exercise of the other residents' rights. Whenever the facility limits such privacy rights, it should document the limitation and the reason for that action in the patient's medical record. The facility should have a written policy governing the limitation of privacy rights.

Federal Laws

Besides the right to privacy found in the federal Constitution and the federal Privacy Act, which applies to the federal government, several federal statutes specify patients' rights to privacy. Section 4211 of Title IV of the Omnibus Budget Reconciliation Act of 1987, Public Law 100-203, detailed patient rights for residents of nursing homes receiving Medicare or Medicaid funds. Among others, patients of such facilities have the right to privacy with regard to accommodations, medical treatment, written and telephonic communications, visits, and meetings of family and of resident groups (42 U.S.C. § 1396r).

State Laws

Alabama

Rules of the Alabama State Board of Health, Division of Licensure and Certification, provide for patient privacy rights in several chapters. Chapter 420-5-7.12(4)(e) requires multipatient hospital bedrooms to have cubicle curtains, screens, or other suitable provisions for privacy. Chapter 420-5-

7.13(1)(c) provides for the segregation of maternity patients in a specifically designated part of the hospital.

Patients of nursing homes have the right to:

- Be treated with consideration, respect, and full consideration of their dignity in caring for personal needs.

- Associate and communicate privately with persons of their choice, and send and receive personal mail unopened, unless medically contraindicated.

- Retain and use personal clothing and possessions as space permits, unless to do so would infringe on the rights of other patients, and unless medically contraindicated.

- If married, have privacy for visits by their spouse. If both are patients, they may share a room, unless medically contraindicated (Rules of Alabama State Board of Health Division of Licensure and Certification, Chapter 420-5-10-.05).

Alaska

Alaska's constitution establishes a right to privacy for its citizens in Alaska Constitution Article 1, § 22. Its administrative code specifies that patients have the right to:

- Associate and communicate privately with persons of their choice.

- Mail and receive unopened correspondence.

- Be treated with consideration and recognition of their dignity and individuality.

- Private visits by their spouses, except in a general acute care hospital, and in a nursing home, to share a room if both spouses are patients in the home, unless medical reasons or space problems require separation (7 Alaska Administrative Code 12.890).

Arizona

Residents of adult care homes have the right, among others, to:

- Be treated with consideration, respect, and full recognition of their dignity and individuality, including the right to privacy in tub, shower, and toilet rooms and in intimate personal hygiene.

- Communicate, associate, and meet privately with persons of their choice in an area provided by the administrator.

- Have access to a telephone, to make and receive calls, and to send and receive correspondence without interception or interference by the owner, manager, or staff of the home (Arizona Revised Statutes § 36-448.08).

Mental health patients, under Arizona Revised Statutes § 36-507, have the right, among others, to:

- Not be fingerprinted.

- Not be photographed without their consent and that of their attorney or guardian, except that patients may be photographed upon admission to an agency for identification and administrative purposes of the agency. All photographs shall be confidential and shall not be released by the agency except pursuant to court order.

Arkansas

Among others, residents of long-term care facilities have the right to:

- Dignity and respect.

- Privacy, including the right to refuse being photographed by persons other than those licensed under the Arkansas Medical Practices Act.

- Personal financial information (Arkansas Statutes § 20-10-1003).

California

Hospitals and medical staffs shall adopt a written policy on patients' rights that provides for, among others:

- Considerate and respectful care.

- Full consideration of privacy concerning the medical care program. Case discussion, consultation, examination, and treatment are confidential and should be conducted discreetly. The patient has the right to be advised about the reason for the presence of any individual.

- Confidential treatment of all communications and records pertaining to the care and the stay in the hospital (22 California Code Regulations § 70707).

Each person involuntarily detained for evaluation or treatment under provisions of this part, each person admitted as a voluntary patient for psychiatric evaluation or treatment to any health facility in which psychiatric evaluation or treatment is offered, and each mentally retarded person committed to a state hospital have the right to:

- See visitors each day.
- Have reasonable access to telephones, both to make and receive confidential calls or to have such calls made for him or her.
- Have ready access to letter-writing materials, including stamps, and to mail and receive unopened correspondence (California Welfare & Institutions Code § 5325).

Each resident of an alcoholism or drug abuse recovery or treatment facility has personal rights that include, but are not limited to, the following:

- The right to confidentiality as provided for in Title 42, Sections 2.1 through 2.67-1, Code of Federal Regulations, effective August 1, 1975.
- Dignity in personal relationships with staff and other persons (9 California Code Regulations § 10569).

Each person with a developmental disability is entitled to the same rights, protections, and responsibilities as all other persons under the laws and Constitution of the State of California, and under the federal laws and the U.S. Constitution. These rights include, but are not limited to:

- Dignity, privacy, and humane care.
- Ability to see visitors each day.
- Reasonable access to telephones, both to make and receive confidential calls and to have calls made for one upon request.
- Freedom to send and receive unopened correspondence and to have ready access to letter-writing materials, including sufficient postage in the form of United States postal stamps (17 California Code Regulations § 50510).

A patient in the comprehensive perinatal services program has the right to be treated with dignity and respect, to have her privacy and confidentiality maintained, among others, under 22 California Code Regulations § 51348.2.

All patients in acute care psychiatric hospitals shall have the right, among others, to:

- See visitors each day.
- Have reasonable access to telephones, both to make and receive confidential calls.

- Have ready access to letter-writing materials, including stamps, and to mail and receive unopened correspondence (22 California Code Regulations § 71507).

Under 22 California Code Regulations § 72453, each patient admitted to a special treatment program in a skilled nursing facility shall have the right to:

- See visitors each day.
- Have reasonable access to telephones, both to make and receive confidential calls.
- Have ready access to letter-writing materials, including stamps, and to mail and receive unopened correspondence.

Patients in skilled nursing facilities have the right of privacy to:

- Manage personal financial affairs or to be given at least a quarterly accounting of financial transactions made on the patient's behalf should the facility accept written delegation of this responsibility.
- Be assured of confidential treatment of financial and health records and to approve or refuse their release, except as authorized by law.
- Be treated with consideration, respect, and full recognition of dignity and individuality, including privacy in treatment and in care of personal needs.
- Associate and communicate privately with persons of the patient's choice, and to send and receive personal mail unopened.
- If married, be assured of privacy for visits by the patient's spouse and if both are patients in the facility, to be permitted to share a room.
- Have visits from members of the clergy at any time at the request of the patient or the patient's representative.
- Have visits from persons of the patient's choosing at any time if the patient is critically ill, unless medically contraindicated.
- Be allowed privacy for visits with family, friends, clergy, social workers, or for professional or business purposes.
- Have reasonable access to telephones and to make and receive confidential calls (22 California Code Regulations § 72527).

Each patient admitted to a special disability program in an intermediate care facility shall have the right, under 22 California Code Regulations § 73399, among others, to:

- Have access to individual storage space for his private use.
- See visitors each day.
- Have reasonable access to telephones, both to make and receive confidential calls.
- Have ready access to letter-writing materials, including stamps, and to mail and receive unopened correspondence.

Intermediate care facility patients shall have the right to:

- Manage personal financial affairs or to be given at least a quarterly accounting of financial transactions made on the patient's behalf should the facility accept his or her written delegation of this responsibility.
- Be assured of confidential treatment of the patient's financial and health records and to approve or refuse their release, by law.
- Be treated with consideration, respect and full recognition of dignity and individuality, including privacy in treatment and in care for personal needs.
- Associate and communicate privately with persons of their choice, and to send and receive personal mail unopened.
- If married, be assured of privacy for visits by their spouse and if both are patients in the facility, to be permitted to share a room.
- Have visits from members of the clergy at the request of the patient or the patient's representative.
- Have visits from persons of their choosing at any time if they are critically ill, unless medically contraindicated.
- Be allowed privacy for visits with family, friends, clergy, social workers, or for professional or business purposes.
- Have reasonable access to telephones both to make and receive confidential calls (22 California Code Regulations 73523).

Among others, clients of home health agencies have the right to be:

- Assured of confidential treatment of personal and medical records and to approve or refuse their release to any individual outside the agency, except in the case of transfer to another health facility, or as required by law or third-party payment contract.

- Treated with consideration, respect, and full recognition of dignity and individuality, including privacy in treatment and in care for personal needs (22 California Code Regulations § 74743).

The governing body of a chemical dependency recovery hospital licensing hospital shall adopt and implement a written policy on patients' rights that must include the right to considerate and respectful care (22 California Code Regulations § 79313).

According to 22 California Code Regulations § 87572, each resident in a residential care facility for the elderly shall have personal rights that include, among others, the right to:

- Be accorded dignity in his or her personal relationships with staff, residents, and other persons.

- Have his or her visitors—including ombudspersons and advocacy representatives—permitted to visit privately during reasonable hours and without prior notice, provided that the rights of other residents are not infringed upon.

- Have access to individual storage space for private use.

- Have reasonable access to telephones, both to make and to receive confidential calls.

- Mail and receive unopened correspondence in a prompt manner.

Each resident of a residential care facility for the chronically ill shall have personal rights under 22 California Code Regulations § 87872 which include, among others, the right to:

- Be accorded dignity in his or her personal relationships with staff and other persons.

- Have access to telephones in order to make and receive confidential calls, provided that such calls do not infringe upon the rights of other residents and do not restrict availability of the telephone during emergencies.

- Mail and receive unopened correspondence in a prompt manner.

Patients in the Alzheimer's Disease Institute demonstration project have, among others, the right to:

- Manage personal financial affairs, or to be given at least a quarterly accounting of financial transactions made on the patient's behalf should the institute accept written delegation of this responsibility.

- Be assured of confidential treatment of personal and medical records and to approve or refuse their release to any individual outside the institute except in the case of transfer to another health facility, or as required by law or this chapter, or by a third-party payment contract.
- Be treated with consideration, respect, and full recognition of dignity and individuality, including privacy in treatment and in care of personal needs.
- Associate and communicate privately with persons of the patient's choice, and to send and receive personal mail unopened, unless medically contraindicated.
- If married, be assured of privacy for visits by the patient's spouse and if both the patients are inpatients, and assigned to the same services unit, to be permitted to share a room, unless medically contraindicated.
- Have daily visiting hours established.
- Have visits from members of the clergy at any time at the request of the patient or the patient's conservator.
- Be allowed privacy for visits with family, friends, clergy, or social workers or for professional or business purposes.
- Have reasonable access to telephones and to make and receive confidential calls (22 California Code Regulations § 97321.29).

Each postsurgical recovery care demonstration project facility shall adopt a written policy on patient rights that must include, among others, rights to:

- Considerate and respectful care.
- Full consideration of privacy concerning the medical care program. Case discussion, consultation, examination, and treatment are confidential and should be conducted discreetly. The patient has the right to be advised of the reason for the presence of any individual (22 California Code Regulations § 97520.15).

Colorado

Patients in nursing facilities have the privacy right to:

- Civil and religious liberties, including knowledge of available choices and the right to independent personal decisions, which will not be infringed upon, and the right to encouragement and assistance from the staff of the facility in the fullest possible exercise of these rights.

- Have private and unrestricted communications with any person of his or her choice.

- Manage his or her own financial affairs or to have a quarterly accounting of any financial transactions made in his or her behalf, should the patient delegate such responsibility to the facility for any period of time.

- Have privacy in treatment and in caring for personal needs, confidentiality in the treatment of personal and medical records, and security in storing and using personal possessions (Colorado Revised Statutes § 25-1-120).

Connecticut

The Patient Bill of Rights for Connecticut healthcare institutions provides, among other rights, that patients:

- May manage personal financial affairs and must be given a quarterly accounting of financial affairs made on their behalf.

- Are assured of confidential treatment of personal and medical records.

- Must receive services with reasonable accommodation of individual needs and preferences, except where the health or safety of the individual would be endangered, and be treated with consideration, respect, and full recognition of their dignity and individuality, including privacy in treatment and care for personal needs.

- May associate and communicate privately with persons of their choice, send and receive personal mail unopened, and make and receive telephone calls privately, unless medically contraindicated.

- Are entitled to organize and participate in patient groups in the facility and to participate in social, religious, and community activities that do not interfere with the rights of other patients, unless medically contraindicated.

- If married, are assured of privacy for visits by their spouses, and if both spouses are inpatients, they are permitted to share a room, unless medically contraindicated (Connecticut General Statutes § 19a-550).

Delaware

Patients in sanatoria, rest homes, nursing homes, boarding homes, and related institutions have the rights, among others, to:

- Be treated with consideration, respect, and full recognition of their dignity and individuality.

- Receive respect and privacy in their medical care program. Case discussion, consultation, examination, and treatment shall be confidential and shall be conducted discreetly. Persons not directly involved in patients' care shall not be permitted to be present during such discussions, consultations, examinations, or treatment.

- Associate and communicate privately and without restriction with persons and groups of their own choice on their own initiative at any reasonable hour; to send and receive mail promptly and unopened; have access at any reasonable hour to a telephone where they may speak privately; and have access to writing instruments, stationery, and postage.

- Manage their own financial affairs. If, by written request signed by the patients and a member of their families or representatives, the facility manages the patients' financial affairs, it shall have available for inspection a monthly accounting, and shall furnish the patients and their families or representatives a quarterly statement of the patients' accounts. The patients and residents shall have unrestricted access to such accounts at reasonable hours.

- If married, enjoy privacy in visits by their spouses, and if both are inpatients of the facility, afforded the opportunity, where feasible, to share a room, unless medically contraindicated.

- Privacy in their rooms, and personnel of the facility shall respect this right by knocking on the door before entering (16 Delaware Code § 1121).

The Mental Health Patients' Bill of Rights adds that each patient is entitled to communicate freely and privately with persons outside the facility as frequently as desired, consistent with the safety and welfare of other patients and with avoiding serious harassment to others. Correspondence initiated to others by the patient shall be sent along promptly without being opened. The hospital shall establish procedures to ensure that patients have full opportunity to conduct correspondence, reasonable access to telephones, and frequent and convenient opportunities to meet with visitors (16 Delaware Code § 5161).

District of Columbia

The District of Columbia Municipal Regulations, Title 22, states, in 3207, that patients have the privacy-related right to:

- Receive visitors privately at any reasonable hour.
- A supportive environment that promotes self-esteem and personal dignity, and protects property and civil rights.
- Receive unopened mail.
- Access to a telephone or to have a private telephone.
- The right of privacy in their rooms. Facility personnel must respect this right by knocking on the door before entering a patient's room.
- If married, privacy for spousal visits. If both spouses are residents, they may share a room unless medically contraindicated.

Florida

Florida law specifies in the Patient's Bill of Rights and Responsibilities that the individual dignity of a patient must be respected at all times and upon all occasions (Florida Statutes § 381.026). The statute adds that every patient who is provided health care retains certain rights to privacy, which providers must respect without regard to the patient's economic status or the source of payment for his or her care. The facility must respect the patient's rights to privacy to the extent consistent with providing adequate medical care to the patient and with the efficient administration of the facility. However, this law does not preclude necessary and discreet discussion of a patient's case or examination by appropriate medical personnel.

Georgia

Under Official Code of Georgia § 31-8-111, each resident of long-term care facilities has the right to associate, meet, and communicate privately with persons of the resident's choice.

Section 31-8-114 specifies such residents' rights to privacy. Each resident shall enjoy the right of privacy, including, but not limited to, the following:

- The right to privacy in the resident's room or the resident's portion of the room. The staff may not enter a resident's room without making their presence known, except when the resident is asleep, in an emergency threatening the health or safety of the resident, or as required by the resident's care plan.

- The right to a private room and a personal sitter if the resident pays the difference between the facility's charge for such a room and sitter and the amount reimbursed through Medicare or Medicaid.

- The right to private visits with the resident's spouse. Spouses shall be permitted to share a room when available where both are residents of the facility.

- The right to have unimpeded, private, and uncensored communication with anyone of the resident's choice by mail, public telephone, and visitation, provided that such visitation does not disturb other residents. The administrator shall provide that mail is received and mailed on regular postal delivery days, that telephones are accessible for confidential and private communications, and that at least one private place per facility is available for visits during normal visitation hours, which shall be for at least 12 continuous hours per day.

- The right to refuse acceptance of correspondence, telephone calls, or visitation by anyone.

- The right to respect and privacy in his or her medical, personal, and bodily care program. Each resident's case discussion, consultation, examination, treatment, and care shall be confidential and shall be conducted in privacy. Those persons not directly involved in the resident's care must have the resident's permission to be present.

- The right to receive confidential treatment of the resident's personal and medical records.

In addition, each resident or his or her guardian shall be permitted to manage the financial affairs of the resident and to withdraw and use funds from any personal account established for him at the facility (*Id.* § 31-8-115). Section 31-8-120 provides for the right of access of visitors.

Under § 37-3-142, mental health patients have the right, among others, to:

- Communicate freely and privately with persons outside the facility and to receive visitors inside the facility.

- Receive and send sealed, unopened mail. No patient's incoming or outgoing mail shall be opened, delayed, held, or censored by the facility. Although this statute has provisions for restricting mail, when warranted, correspondence of the patient with his or her attorney or with public officials shall not be restricted in any manner.

Section 37-3-160 requires respect for the individual dignity of mental health patients, and § 37-3-163 requires respect for bodily integrity.

Under § 37-7-142, each patient in a facility for the treatment of alcoholism or drug dependency or abuse shall have the right to communicate freely and privately with persons outside the facility and to receive visitors inside the facility. With some restrictions, such as if reasonable grounds exist to believe the mail contains dangerous materials, each patient shall be allowed to receive and send sealed, unopened mail; no patient's incoming or outgoing mail shall be opened, delayed, held, or censored by the facility. Again, the facility may not restrict correspondence with the patient's attorney or with public officials. Under § 37-7-160, such patient's individual dignity must be preserved; his or her bodily integrity must also be preserved, according to § 37-7-163. Subject to reasonable rules regarding hours of visitation that the commissioner may adopt, patients in any approved treatment facility shall be granted opportunities for adequate consultation with counsel and for continuing contact with family and friends consistent with an effective treatment program (*Id.* § 37-8-51).

Chapter 290-5-6.14, Rules and Regulations for Hospitals, Georgia Department of Human Resources, specifies that fire-resistant cubicle curtains, adequate to allow privacy, shall be available for use in rooms occupied by more than one patient to allow for privacy of each patient without obstructing the passage for the other patient either to the corridor or to the toilet or lavatory adjacent to the patient's room. This requirement is optional for hospitals providing care for psychiatric, alcoholic, and mentally retarded patients.

Hawaii

Patients in Hawaiian facilities have the right, among others, to:

- Be treated with consideration and respect and in full recognition of their dignity and individuality.

- Associate and communicate privately with persons of their choice, and to send and receive their personal mail unopened.

- Be assured of privacy for visits. If spouses are both patients in a facility, they are permitted to share a room.

- Manage their personal financial affairs (Administrative Rule, Title 11, Chapter 94, § 26, Patient's Rights).

Mental health services patients have the rights to privacy, respect, and personal dignity and to visitation rights unless the patient poses a danger to self or others. However, if the facility prohibits visitation, it must allow the legal guardians or legal representatives to visit the patients on request (Hawaii Revised Statutes § 334E-2). Patients also have the right to uncensored communications (*Id).*

Idaho

A residential care facility must protect and promote the rights of each resident, including each of the following rights, among others, under Idaho Code § 39-3316:

- Each resident must be assured of the right to privacy with regard to accommodations, medical and other treatment, written and telephone communications, visits, and meetings of family and resident groups.
- Each resident shall have the right to be treated with dignity and respect.
- Each facility must permit:
  - Immediate access to a resident, subject to the resident's right to deny or withdraw consent at any time, by immediate family or other relatives.
  - Immediate access to a resident, subject to reasonable restrictions and the resident's right to deny or withdraw consent at any time, by others who are visiting with the consent of the resident.
  - Reasonable access to a resident by any entity or individual that provides health, social, legal, or other services to the resident, subject to the resident's right to deny or withdraw consent at any time.
- Each resident shall have the right to confidentiality of personal and clinical records.

A residential care facility for the elderly must protect and promote the rights of each resident, under Idaho Code § 39-3516, including the right to:

- Privacy with regard to accommodations, medical and other treatment, written and telephone communications, visits, and meetings of family and resident groups.
- Be treated with dignity and respect.
- Access and visitation. Each facility must permit:
  - Immediate access to any resident by any representative of the department, by the state ombudsman for the elderly or his or her designee, or by the resident's individual physician.

- Immediate access to a resident, subject to the resident's right to deny or withdraw consent at any time, by immediate family or other relatives.

- Immediate access to a resident, subject to reasonable restrictions and the resident's right to deny or withdraw consent at any time, by others who are visiting with the consent of the resident.

- Reasonable access to a resident by any entity or individual that provides health, social, legal, or other services to the resident, subject to the resident's right to deny or withdraw consent at any time.

- Confidentiality of personal and clinical records.

- Confidentiality and privacy concerning his or her medical or dental condition and treatment.

Under § 39-3387, residents of adult foster care homes have the same rights.

Every patient hospitalized for mental illness shall have the right to:

- Communicate by sealed mail or otherwise with persons inside or outside the facility and have access to reasonable amounts of letter-writing material and postage.

- Receive visitors at all reasonable times.

- Refuse specific modes of treatment.

- Be visited by his or her attorney at all times (Idaho Code § 66-346).

Home health agencies must afford patients' rights as specified for the Medicare and Medicaid programs (*Id.* § 39-2409).

Illinois

The Medical Patients Rights Act establishes the right of patients to privacy and confidentiality in health care (410 Illinois Compiled Statutes 50/3).

A nursing home resident has the right, among others, to:

- Manage his or her own personal affairs (210 ILCS 45/2-102).

- Respect and privacy in medical and personal care programs. Every resident's case discussion, consultation, examination, and treatment shall be confidential and shall be conducted discreetly. Those persons not directly involved in the resident's care must have his or her permission to be present (*Id.* 45/2-105).

- Unimpeded, private, and uncensored communication of his or her choice by mail, public telephone, or visitation. The administrator must ensure that residents may have private visits at any reasonable hour unless not medically advisable. The administrator must also ensure that married residents residing in the same facility are allowed to reside in the same room unless no room is available or it is medically inadvisable (*Id.* 45/2-108).

Indiana

Health facility residents have the right, among others, to:

- Be treated with consideration, respect, and recognition of their dignity and individuality.
- Be afforded confidentiality of treatment.
- When both husband and wife are residents in the facility, live as a family in a suitable room or quarters, if practical, and to occupy a double bed unless medically contraindicated.
- Be treated as individuals with consideration and respect for their privacy. The facility shall afford privacy for at least the following:
  - Bathing.
  - Personal care.
  - Physical examinations and treatments.
  - Visitations.
  - Choose with whom they will associate. The facility shall have reasonable visiting hours.
  - Receive intact and unopened mail (410 Indiana Administrative Code 16.2-2-3).

The rules for hospitals provide that such facilities must provide visual privacy for patients in multibed rooms (410 IAC 15-1-10).

Indiana Code § 12-27-3-1 adds that individuals being treated for mental illness or developmental disabilities have the rights to:

- Be visited at reasonable times.
- Send and receive sealed mail.
- Have access to a reasonable amount of letter-writing materials and postage.
- Place and receive telephone calls at the patient's own expense.

Community residential facilities for persons with developmental disabilities must contain sufficient living areas in addition to bedrooms for the comfort and privacy of residents (431 IAC 1.1-3-7).

Residents of community residential facilities for the mentally ill have the right, among others, to:

- Be treated with consideration, respect, and full recognition of their dignity and individuality.
- Communicate, associate, and meet privately with persons of their choice.
- Have access in reasonable privacy to a telephone.
- Send and receive mail unopened.
- Privacy of self and possessions.
- Manage personal financial affairs or to seek assistance in managing them (431 IAC 2-2-4).

Such facilities must have sufficient living areas in addition to bedrooms for the comfort and privacy of residents (431 IAC 2-2-8).

Iowa

Hospital governing boards must adopt principles regarding patient rights that must address, among others, preservation of individual dignity and protection of personal privacy in the receipt of care [Iowa Administrative Code 481-51.5(135B)].

The Iowa Administrative Code Rules Setting Minimum Standards for Intermediate Care Facilities specifies, in Chapter 58, as does Minimum Standards for Nursing Facilities in Chapter 59, that residents shall be treated with consideration, respect, and full recognition of their dignity and individuality, including privacy in treatment and in care for their personal needs [481-58.45(135C) and 481-59.50(135C)]. Residents shall be examined and treated in a manner that maintains the privacy of their bodies. A closed door or a drawn curtain shall shield the resident from passersby. Any person not involved in the care of the residents shall not be present without the residents' consent while they are being examined or treated. Privacy of residents' bodies also shall be maintained during toileting, bathing, and other activities of personal hygiene, except as needed for resident safety or assistance. Staff shall knock and be acknowledged before entering a resident's room unless the resident is not capable of a response. This rule does not apply in emergency conditions. These rules also provide that residents may communicate, associate, and meet privately with persons of their choice (unless to do so would infringe on the rights of other residents) and may send and receive personal mail unopened. Residents may also receive visits from anyone they wish, subject to reasonable scheduling restrictions, and may make and receive telephone calls with privacy (*Id*).

Kansas

Adult care homes in Kansas must ensure that residents have the right, among others, to:

- Be treated with consideration, respect, and full recognition of dignity and individuality, including privacy in treatment and in care for personal needs.

- Be permitted to associate and communicate privately with persons of their choice and to send and receive personal mail unopened, unless medically contraindicated.

- If married, be assured of privacy for visits by their spouse. If both are residents of the facility, they shall be permitted to share the same room unless medically contraindicated (Kansas Administrative Regulations § 28-39-78).

Kentucky

Under Kentucky Revised Statutes § 216.515, residents of long-term care facilities have, among others, the right to:

- Manage the use of their personal funds.

- If married, be assured of privacy for the spouse's visits and if they are both residents in the facility, share the same room unless they are in different levels of care or unless medically contraindicated and documented by a physician in the resident's medical record.

- Associate and communicate privately with persons of their choice and send and receive personal mail unopened.

- Be assured of at least visual privacy in multibed rooms and in tub, shower, and toilet rooms.

- Be treated with consideration, respect, and full recognition of their dignity and individuality, including privacy in treatment and in care for their personal needs.

- Be suitably dressed at all times and given assistance when needed in maintaining body hygiene and good grooming.

- Have access to a telephone at a convenient location within the facility for making and receiving telephone calls.

- Have private meetings with the appropriate long-term care facility inspectors from the Cabinet for Human Resources.

Every resident in a boarding home has the right, among others, to:

- Manage the use of his or her personal funds.

- Associate and communicate privately with persons of his or her choice, within reasonable hours established by the boarding home, and send and receive personal mail unopened.

- Be assured of at least visual privacy in multibed rooms and in bathrooms.

- Be treated with consideration, respect, and full recognition of his or her dignity and individuality.

- Have access to a telephone at a convenient location within the boarding home for making and receiving telephone calls subject to reasonable rules established by the boarding home.

- Have private meetings with inspectors representing the Cabinet for Human Resources (Kentucky Revised Statutes § 216B.303).

Louisiana

Title 40, Public Safety, Chapter 11, State Department of Hospitals Residents' Bill of Rights, 40 Louisiana Revised Statutes § 2010.8, specifies that nursing home residents have the right, among others, to:

- Private and uncensored communications, including but not limited to receiving and sending unopened correspondence; access to a telephone; visitation with any person of their choice; and overnight visitation outside the facility with family and friends in accordance with pertinent laws, regulations, and nursing home policies.

- Manage their own financial affairs or to delegate such responsibility to the nursing home.

- Privacy in treatment and in caring for personal needs; have closed room doors; and have facility personnel knock before entering the room, except in case of an emergency or unless medically contraindicated. Privacy of the resident's body shall be maintained during, but not limited to, toileting, bathing, and other activities of personal hygiene, except as needed for resident safety or assistance.

Maine

Under 5 Maine Revised Statutes § 20048, subject to reasonable rules regarding hours of visitation that the director may adopt, patients in any approved substance abuse treatment facility must be granted opportunities for adequate consultation with counsel and for continuing contact with family and friends consistent with an effective treatment program. Mail or other communication to or from a patient in any approved treatment facility may not be intercepted, read, or censored. The director may adopt reasonable rules regarding the use of telephones by patients in approved treatment facilities.

A patient in a hospital or residential care facility for mental health treatment has the right, among others under 34-B Maine Revised Statutes § 3803, to:

- Communicate by sealed envelopes with the department, a member of the clergy of his or her choice, his or her attorney, and the court that ordered the hospitalization, if any.
- Communicate by mail in accordance with the rules of the hospital.
- Receive visitors unless definitely contraindicated by his or her medical condition, except that he or she may be visited by a member of the clergy of his or her choice or attorney at any reasonable time.

Maryland

The Maryland General Assembly has established a state policy, in Maryland Health-General Code § 19-343, that each resident of a comprehensive care or extended care facility has the right, among others, to:

- Be treated with consideration, respect, and full recognition of human dignity and individuality.
- Privacy.
- Receive respect and privacy in a medical care program.
- Manage personal financial affairs.

Massachusetts

Under Massachusetts Laws Chapter 111, § 70E, patients have the right to privacy during medical treatment or other rendering of care within the capacity of the facility. Every patient or resident of a facility shall be provided by the physician in the facility the right to:

- Privacy during medical treatment or other rendering of care within the capacity of the facility.

- Refuse to be examined, observed, or treated by students or any other facility staff without jeopardizing access to psychiatric, psychological, or other medical care and attention.

Patients in drug facilities have the right to have a physician retained by them examine them, to consult privately with their attorney, to receive visitors, and to send and receive communications by mail, telephone, and telegraph. Such communications shall not be censored or read without the consent of such patients. The foregoing shall not limit the right of the administrator, subject to reasonable rules and regulations of the division, to prescribe reasonable rules governing visiting hours and the use of telephone and telegraph facilities (Massachusetts Laws chapter 111E, § 18).

Any mentally ill person in the care of the department under the provisions of this chapter shall be provided with stationery and postage in reasonable amounts and shall have the right to have letters forwarded unopened to the governor, to the commissioner, to his or her personal physician, attorney, clergy, to any court, to any publicly elected official, and to any member of his or her immediate family. The superintendent may open and restrict the forwarding of any other letters written by said person when in said person's best interest (Massachusetts Laws chapter 123, § 23). A mentally ill person has the right to be visited at all reasonable times by his or her personal physician, attorney, and clergy, and the right to be visited by other persons unless the superintendent determines that such a visit by any of said persons would not be in the best interest of the mentally ill person and incorporates a statement of the reasons for any denial of visiting rights in the treatment record of said person.

Under the Ombudsman Program Statute (*Id.* chapter 19A, § 29), the ombudsman—or any designated local ombudsman program or representative of a community group offering legal services or free advocacy assistance, certified by the secretary of the department of elder affairs—shall be permitted access at reasonable hours. The person or representative shall have the right to visit privately with the resident only after the resident has given permission for such visit; shall, at all times, respect the confidentiality of all such communications; and shall not subject the resident to photographing, filming, videotaping, or audiotaping without written permission of the resident or his or her legal representative.

Michigan

The Michigan Public Health Code prescribes the right of patients or residents, among others, to:

- Privacy, to the extent feasible, in treatment and caring for personal needs with consideration, respect, and full recognition of their dignity and individuality.

- Associate and have private communications and consultations with their physicians, attorneys, or any other persons of their choice and to send and receive personal mail unopened on the same day it is received, unless medically contraindicated.

- Associate and communicate privately with persons of their own choice. Facilities must afford reasonable privacy for visitation of a patient who shares a room with another patient. A married nursing home patient or home for the aged resident is entitled to meet privately with his or her spouse in a room that ensures privacy. If both spouses are residents in the same facility, they are entitled to share a room unless medically contraindicated (Michigan Compiled Laws § 333.20201).

Minnesota

Minnesota's Patients and Residents of Health Care Facilities Bill of Rights states that patients and residents have the right to be treated with courtesy and respect for their individuality by employees of or persons providing service in a healthcare facility. It adds that they also have the right to respectfulness and privacy within their medical and personal care program. Case discussion, consultation, examination, and treatment are confidential and shall be conducted discreetly. Providers shall respect privacy during toileting, bathing, and other activities of personal hygiene, except as needed for patient or resident safety or assistance. Patients and residents also have the right to every consideration of their privacy, individuality, and cultural identity as related to their social, religious, and psychological well-being. Facility staff shall respect the privacy of a resident's room by knocking on the door and seeking consent before entering, except in an emergency or where clearly inadvisable (Minnesota Statutes § 144.651).

Mississippi

A mentally ill or mentally retarded patient has the right to correspond freely without censorship. The director of the treatment facility may restrict receipt of correspondence if the director determines that the medical welfare of the patient requires it. No restriction shall be placed upon correspondence between a patient and his or her attorney or any court of competent jurisdiction (Mississippi Code § 41-21-102). Subject to the general rules of the treatment facility, a patient has the right to receive visitors and make phone calls. The director of the treatment facility may restrict visits and phone calls if he or she determines that the medical welfare of the patient requires it. No restriction shall be placed upon a patient's visitation at the treatment facility with or upon calls to or from his or her attorney.

A patient has the right to meet with or call his or her personal physician, spiritual advisor, and counsel at all reasonable times *(Id)*.

Missouri

Residents in long-term care facilities have certain rights under Missouri's Long-Term Care Facility Regulations and Licensure Law for Residential Care Facilities I and II, Intermediate Care Facilities, and Skilled Nursing Facilities (13 CSR 15-18.010). Among others, these rights include the following:

- Residents shall be treated with consideration, respect, and full recognition of their dignity, individuality, and privacy in treatment and care of personal needs. All persons, other than the attending physician, the facility personnel necessary for any treatment or personal care, or the Division of Aging or Department of Mental Health staff, as appropriate, shall be excluded from observing residents during any time of examination, treatment, or care unless residents consent.

- Residents may communicate, associate, and meet privately with others of their choice unless to do so would infringe upon the rights of other residents. The facility must permit residents to meet alone with persons of their choice and provide an area that ensures privacy.

- Telephones shall be accessible at all times to residents to make and receive calls, and privacy shall be provided when possible.

- If residents cannot open mail, the facility shall obtain written consent to open mail and read it to the residents.

- Married residents shall be assured of privacy for visits by their spouses. When spouses visit and request privacy, the room will be provided with a sign for the door visibly stating "Private—Do Not Enter." If the married couple's door is closed, personnel must knock and wait for invitation to enter. If no response is given, staff shall be permitted to enter the room.

- If both husband and wife are residents, they shall be allowed the choice of sharing a room.

Mental health patients have the right to communicate by sealed mail or otherwise, to have reasonable access to a telephone to make and receive confidential calls, and to receive visits from their attorney, physician, or clergy, in private, at reasonable times (Revised Statutes of Missouri § 630.110).

Montana

Under Montana Code § 50-5-1104, long-term care facility residents have the rights applied by the federal government to facilities that provide skilled nursing care or intermediate nursing care and participate in a Medicaid or Medicare program [42 U.S.C. 1395x(j) and 1396d(c)], as implemented by regulation. In addition, residents have the right to privacy in their rooms or portions of the room. If residents seek privacy in their rooms, staff members should make reasonable efforts to make their presence known when entering.

Under Montana Code §53-20-142, developmentally disabled persons admitted to a residential facility for a period of habilitation shall enjoy the right, among others, to:

- Dignity, privacy, and humane care.

- Send and receive sealed mail. Moreover, it is the duty of the facility to foster the exercise of this right by furnishing the necessary materials and assistance.

- Private telephone communication as do patients at any public hospital, except to the extent that the individual treatment planning team or the qualified professional responsible for formulation of a particular resident's habilitation plan writes an order imposing special restrictions and explains the reasons for the restrictions.

- Visitation except to the extent that the individual treatment planning team or the qualified professional responsible for formulation of a particular resident's habilitation plan writes an order imposing special restrictions and explains the reasons for the restrictions.

- Under appropriate supervision, to suitable opportunities for the interaction with members of the opposite sex except where the individual treatment planning team or the qualified professional

responsible for the formulation of a particular resident's habilitation plan writes an order to the contrary and explains the reasons
for the order.

Under Montana Code § 53-21-142, patients admitted to a mental
health facility, whether voluntarily or involuntarily, shall have the right,
among others, to:

- Privacy and dignity.

- Visitation and reasonable access to telephone communications, including the right to converse with others privately, except to the
  extent that the professional person responsible for formulation of
  a particular patient's treatment plan writes an order imposing special restrictions. Patients shall have an unrestricted right to visitation with attorneys, spiritual counselors, private physicians, and
  other professional persons.

- Send sealed mail unrestricted. Patients shall have an unrestricted
  right to receive sealed mail from their attorneys, private physicians,
  and other professional persons, the mental disabilities board of visitors, courts, and government officials. Patients shall have a right to
  receive sealed mail from others except to the extent that a professional person responsible for formulation of the patients' treatment
  plan writes an order imposing special restrictions on receipt of
  sealed mail.

- Access to letter-writing materials, including postage, and have a
  right to have staff members of the facility assist persons who are
  unable to write, prepare, and mail correspondence.

- Be provided, with adequate supervision, suitable opportunities for
  interaction with members of the opposite sex except to the extent
  that a professional person in charge of the patients' treatment plan
  writes an order stating that such interaction is inappropriate to the
  treatment regimen.

- A humane psychological and physical environment within the
  mental health facilities. These facilities shall be designed to afford patients with comfort and safety, promote dignity, and ensure privacy.

Subject to reasonable rules regarding hours of visitation that the department may adopt, patients in any approved alcoholism treatment facility
shall be granted opportunities for adequate consultation with counsel and
for continuing contact with family and friends consistent with an effective
treatment program. Neither mail nor other communication to or from a

patient in any approved treatment facility may be intercepted, read, or censored. The administrator may adopt reasonable rules regarding the use of telephone by patients in approved treatment facilities (Montana Code § 53-24-305).

Nebraska

Among others, residents of skilled nursing facilities have the right to:

- Manage their own personal financial affairs.
- Be treated with consideration, respect, and full recognition of their dignity and individuality, including privacy in treatment and in care for personal needs. Residents must be examined and treated in a way that maintains the privacy of their bodies.
- A closed door or drawn curtain to shield the resident from passers-by. People not involved in the care of the residents must not be present without the residents' consent while they are being examined or treated.
- Privacy of their bodies during toileting, bathing, and other activities of personal hygiene, except as needed for resident safety or assistance.
- Communicate, associate, and meet privately with persons of their own choice, unless to do so would infringe on the rights of other residents.
- Send and receive personal mail unopened.
- Have facility personnel identify themselves and receive permission before entering residents' immediate living areas.
- Receive visitors in reasonable comfort and privacy.
- Privacy for visits by spouses. If both are residents, the facility shall permit them to share a room. The facility must have a method of arranging privacy in visits between spouses (Title 175, Chapter 12, Regulations and Standards for Skilled Nursing Facilities 003.02).

Nevada

Every patient of a medical facility or facility for the dependent has the rights, among others, to retain his or her privacy concerning a program of medical care. Discussions of a patient's care, consultation with other persons concerning the patient, examinations or treatments, and all communications and records concerning the patient are confidential. The patient must consent to the presence of any person who is not directly involved in his or her care during any examination, consultation, or treatment (Nevada Revised Statutes § 449.720).

New Hampshire

The New Hampshire Residential Care and Health Facility Licensing Patients' Bill of Rights, New Hampshire Revised Statutes 151:21, requires such facilities to have policies:

- Permitting patients to manage their own personal financial affairs.
- Ensuring confidential treatment of all information in patients' personal or clinical records.
- Specifying that patients are free to communicate with, associate with, and meet privately with anyone, unless to do so would infringe on the rights of other patients.
- Permitting patients to send and receive unopened mail and to have regular access to the unmonitored use of a telephone.
- Permitting patients to participate in social, religious, and community group activities, unless to do so would infringe upon the rights of other patients.
- Requiring privacy for visits and permitting married patients to share rooms with the other spouse unless medically contraindicated.

The Home Care Client's Bill of Rights requires home healthcare providers to treat clients with consideration, respect, and full recognition of the client's dignity and individuality, including privacy in treatment and personal care and respect for personal property (Revised Statutes 151:21-b).

New Jersey

New Jersey's Bill of Rights for hospital patients, New Jersey Statutes § 26:2H-12.8, specifies that every person admitted to a general hospital as licensed by the State Department of Health shall have the right to privacy to the extent consistent with providing adequate medical care to the patient. This shall not preclude discussion of a patient's case or examination of a patient by appropriate healthcare personnel.

Patients hospitalized for mental illness have, among others, the right to:

- Privacy and dignity.
- See visitors each day.

- Have reasonable access to and use of telephones, both to make and receive confidential calls.

- Have ready access to letter-writing materials, including stamps, and to mail and receive unopened correspondence.

- Suitable opportunities for interaction with members of the opposite sex, with adequate supervision (*Id.* § 30:4-27.2).

A psychiatric patient receiving treatment in a short-term care facility shall have the right to:

- Privacy and dignity.

- See visitors each day.

- Have reasonable access to and use of telephones, both to make and receive confidential calls.

- Have ready access to letter-writing materials, including stamps, and to mail and receive unopened correspondence.

- Suitable opportunities for interaction with members of the opposite sex, with adequate supervision (*Id.* § 30:4-27.11d).

Under New Jersey Statutes § 30:13-5, every resident of a nursing home shall have the right to:

- Manage his or her own financial affairs unless the resident or his or her guardian authorizes the administrator of the nursing home to manage such resident's financial affairs.

- Receive and send unopened correspondence and, upon request, to obtain assistance in the reading and writing of such correspondence.

- Unaccompanied access to a telephone at a reasonable hour, including the right to a private phone at the resident's expense.

- Privacy.

- Unrestricted communication, including personal visitation with any persons of his or her choice, at any reasonable hour.

- Reasonable opportunity for interaction with members of the opposite sex. If married, the resident shall enjoy reasonable privacy in visits by his or her spouse and, if both are residents of the nursing home, they shall be afforded the opportunity, where feasible, to share a room, unless medically inadvisable.

New Mexico

Aside from the confidentiality of medical information, the *New Mexico Hospital Association Handbook* suggests that hospitals establish policies governing the circumstances under which patients may be photographed by the media, the facility, law enforcement personnel, or attorneys. Such policies should require the patient, his or her legal representative, or the attending physician to consent to any request to have photographs taken of the patient, unless the photograph is needed for law enforcement purposes where the consenting party is a major suspect, such as in a child abuse investigation (*Id.* chapter 3.H).

New York

All patients in New York medical facilities have the right, among others, to:

- No infringement of civil and religious liberties, including the right to independent personal decisions and knowledge of available choices.

- Private communications and consultations with their physician, attorney, and any other person.

- Manage their own financial affairs, or to have at least a quarterly accounting of any personal financial transactions undertaken on their behalf by the facility during any period of time the patient has delegated such responsibilities to the facility.

- Privacy in treatment and in caring for personal needs (New York Consolidated Laws Service Public Health § 2803-c).

North Carolina

The Nursing Home Patients' Bill of Rights specifies that every patient has the right, among others, to:

- Be treated with consideration, respect, and full recognition of personal dignity and individuality.

- Receive respect and privacy in the patient's medical care program. Case discussion, consultation, examination, and treatment shall remain confidential and shall be conducted discreetly.

- Associate and communicate privately and without restriction with persons and groups of the patient's choice on the patient's initiative or that of the persons or groups at any reasonable hour; to send and receive mail promptly and unopened, unless the patient is unable to open and read personal mail; to have access at any reasonable hour to a telephone where the patient may speak privately; and to have access to writing instruments, stationery, and postage.

- Manage the patient's financial affairs unless authority has been properly delegated to another or another has been appointed pursuant to law.

- Enjoy privacy in visits by his or her spouse, and if both are inpatients of the facility, they shall be afforded the opportunity, where feasible, to share a room.

- Enjoy privacy in the patient's room (North Carolina General States § 131E-117).

North Dakota

North Dakota healthcare facility residents have, among others, the right to:

- Have private meetings, associations, and communications with any person of the residents' choice within the facility.

- Send and receive unopened personal mail and the right of access to and use of telephones for private conversations.

- Be assured of private visits by their spouse, or if both are residents of the same facility, the right to share a room, unless such is not medically advisable.

- Manage their own financial affairs if not under legal guardianship, or to delegate that responsibility in writing.

- Have privacy in treatment and in caring for personal needs.

- Be treated courteously, fairly, and with the fullest measure of dignity (North Dakota Century Code § 50-10.2-02).

Mentally ill and retarded patients in treatment facilities for such conditions have the rights to be treated with dignity and respect, to visitation and telephone communications, and to send and receive sealed mail (*Id.* § 25-03.1-40).

Ohio

Ohio Revised Code § 3721.13 contains one of the most detailed listings of patient rights. Under it, the residents of a rest or nursing home shall have, but are not limited to, the right to:

- Be treated at all times with courtesy, respect, and full recognition of dignity and individuality.

- Confidential treatment of personal and medical records.

- Privacy during medical examination or treatment and in the care of personal or bodily needs.

- Consume a reasonable amount of alcoholic beverages at their own expense, unless not medically advisable as documented in his medical record by the attending physician or unless contradictory to written admission policies.

- Use tobacco at their own expense under the home's safety rules and under applicable laws and rules of the state, unless not medically advisable as documented in their medical records by the attending physicians or unless contradictory to written admission policies.

- Retire and rise in accordance with their reasonable requests, if they do not disturb others or the posted meal schedules and upon the home's request remain in a supervised area, unless not medically advisable as documented by the attending physician.

- Upon reasonable request, have private and unrestricted communications with their families, social workers, and any other person, unless not medically advisable as documented in their medical record by the attending physician, except that communications with public officials or with his attorney or physician shall not be restricted. Private and unrestricted communications shall include, but are not limited to, the right to:

  - Send, and mail sealed, unopened correspondence.

  - Access to a telephone for private communications.

  - Visits at any reasonable hour.

- Be assured of privacy for visits by their spouse, or if both are residents of the same home, the right to share a room within the capacity of the home, unless not medically advisable as documented in their medical record by the attending physician.

- Upon reasonable request, have room doors closed and to have them not opened without knocking, except in the case of an emergency or unless not medically advisable as documented in their medical record by the attending physician.

- Manage their personal financial affairs, or, if patients delegate this responsibility in writing to the home, to receive upon written request at least a quarterly accounting statement of financial transactions made on their behalf.

Section 3722.12 governs rights of residents of adult care facilities. Among others, those include the right to:

- Be treated at all times with courtesy and respect, and with full recognition of personal dignity and individuality.
- Practice a religion of their choice or to abstain from the practice of religion.
- Manage personal financial affairs.
- Engage in or refrain from engaging in activities of their own choosing within reason.
- Private and unrestricted communications, including the right to:
  - Receive, send, and mail sealed, unopened correspondence.
  - Reasonable access to a telephone for private communications.
  - Private visits at any reasonable hour.
- Share a room with a spouse if both are residents of the facility.

Rights of residents of community alternative homes include, among others, the right to:

- Be treated at all times with courtesy, respect, and full recognition of personal dignity and individuality.
- Privacy during medical examination or treatment and in the care of personal or bodily needs.
- Retire and rise in accordance with his or her reasonable request, if they do not disturb others or interfere with meal schedules.
- Observe religious obligations and participate in religious activities.
- Manage personal financial affairs.
- Engage in activities of their own choosing within reason, or to refrain from engaging in activities.
- Private and unrestricted communications, including:
  - Receiving and sending sealed, unopened correspondence.
  - Reasonable access to a telephone for private communications.
  - Private visits at a reasonable hour (*Id.* § 3724.07).

Under § 5122.29, patients hospitalized for mental illness have the right, among others, to:

- Be treated at all times with consideration and respect for their privacy and dignity.

- Communicate freely with and be visited at reasonable times by their private counsel or personnel of the legal rights service and, unless prior court restriction has been obtained, to communicate freely with and be visited at reasonable times by their personal physician or psychologist.

- Communicate freely with others, unless specifically restricted in the patients' treatment plans for clear treatment reasons, including without limitation the following:

  - Receive visitors at reasonable times.

  - Have reasonable access to telephones to make and receive confidential calls, including a reasonable number of free calls if unable to pay for them and assistance in calling if requested and needed.

  - Have ready access to letter-writing materials, including a reasonable number of stamps without cost if unable to pay for them, and to mail and receive unopened correspondence and assistance in writing if requested and needed.

- Receive and possess reading materials without censorship, except when the materials create a clear and present danger to the safety of persons in the facility.

- Reasonable privacy, including both periods of privacy and places of privacy.

Oklahoma

Under the Nursing Home Care Act, residents have the right, among others, to:

- Have private communications, including telephone communications and visits and consultation with the physician, attorney, meetings of family and resident groups or any other person of their choice, and to send and promptly receive, unopened, their personal mail.

- Manage their own financial affairs, unless the residents delegate the responsibility, in writing, to the facility.

- Receive respect and privacy in their medical care program. Case discussion, consultation, examination, and treatment shall remain confidential and shall be conducted discreetly.

- Privacy for spousal visits. Residents may share a room with their spouse, if married and the spouse is residing in the same facility (63 Oklahoma Statutes § 1-1918).

Residents of group homes for the developmentally disabled or physically handicapped have essentially the same rights under 63 Oklahoma Statutes § 1-818.20.

Patients at institutions for the care and treatment of mental health patients have the privilege of freely writing to and corresponding by uncensored and sealed letter mail, which is either sent out or received, with their relatives, friends, physicians, and legal advisers. They may also receive visits from those persons at reasonable times and have reasonable telephone privileges, except when the institution's administrator deems it inadvisable and documents the reason in the patient's clinical case record.

However, notwithstanding any such limitations, all patients are entitled to communicate at all times by uncensored sealed letter mail with official agencies, the court that ordered their commitment, and their personal attorney and physician (43A Oklahoma Statutes § 4-107).

Oregon

Nursing home residents have the right to be treated with respect and dignity and to be assured of complete privacy during treatment and when receiving personal care under the Nursing Home Patients' Bill of Rights. They also have the right to:

- Manage personal finances or be given a quarterly report of account if the facility has been delegated in writing to carry out this responsibility.

- Associate and communicate privately with persons of the residents' choice and send and receive personal mail unopened unless medically contraindicated.

- Participate in activities of social, religious, and community groups at their discretion unless medically contraindicated.

- If married, privacy for visits by their spouse. If both spouses are residents in a facility, they are permitted to share a room (Oregon Revised Statutes § 441.605).

Pennsylvania

Pennsylvania law, in 35 Pennsylvania Statutes § 448.801a, which governs the licensing of healthcare facilities, states that one of the purposes of the licensing laws is to ensure quality health care through appropriate and nonduplicative review and inspection with due regard to the protection of the health and rights of privacy of patients and without unreasonably interfering with the operation of the healthcare facility or home health agency. 28 Pennsylvania Administrative Code § 103.22 requires hospital governing bodies to establish patient bills of rights not less in substance or coverage than the minimum rights enumerated in the code. Among those rights are the right to every consideration of a patient's privacy concerning his or her own medical care program. Case discussion, consultation, examination, and treatment are considered confidential and should be conducted discreetly (*Id*).

Patients of long-term nursing homes have the right, among others, to:

- Manage their own personal financial affairs.

- Be treated with consideration, respect, and full recognition of dignity and individuality, including privacy in treatment and in care for their necessary personal and social needs.

- Be permitted to associate and communicate privately with persons of choice. Patients shall be permitted to send and receive personal mail unopened. Facility staff may assist patients in sending or receiving personal mail if patients request assistance.

- Meet in private with visitors or persons of their choice (28 Pennsylvania Code § 201.29).

Birth centers must have policies that assure the individual mother the right to dignity, privacy, and safety, including confidentiality, anonymity, and privacy (28 Pennsylvania Code § 501.46).

Adults in residential agencies, facilities, and services have the right to:

- Privacy of self and possessions.

- Associate and communicate with others privately.

- Access in reasonable privacy to a telephone in the home and make local calls without charge, except where a standard pay telephone is used.

- Access the U.S. mail, and write and send mail, at the residents' own expense, and receive uncensored and unopened mail.

- Be treated with dignity and respect (55 Pennsylvania Code § 2620.61).

Mental health patients have the right, among others, to:

- Unrestricted and private communication inside and outside the facility.

- Receive visitors of their own choice at reasonable hours unless a treatment team has determined in advance that a visitor or visitors would seriously interfere with their or others' treatment or welfare.

- Receive and send unopened letters and to have outgoing letters stamped and mailed. Incoming mail may be examined for good reason in the patient's presence for contraband. *Contraband* means specific property that threatens patients' health and welfare or the hospital community's.
- Have access to telephone designated for patient use.
- Handle their personal affairs (55 Pennsylvania Code § 5100.53).

Rhode Island

Rhode Island's laws governing the licensing of healthcare facilities, Rhode Island General Laws § 23-17-19.1, specify that patients shall be afforded considerate and respectful care and that the right to privacy shall be respected to the extent consistent with providing adequate medical care to the patient and with the efficient administration of the healthcare facility. Nothing in this statute, however, precludes discreet discussion of patients' cases or examination of appropriate medical personnel.

Residents of residential care/assisted living facilities for adults have the right, among others, to:

- Be cared for with consideration, respect, and dignity.
- Be afforded their rights to freedom of religious practice, civil liberties, maintenance of self-independence, and privacy.
- Associate and communicate privately with persons of their choice and be allowed freedom and privacy in sending and receiving mail.
- Manage their own personal financial affairs (*Id.* § 23-17.4-16).

Nursing home patients shall be treated and cared for with consideration, respect, and dignity, and shall be afforded their right to privacy to the extent consistent with providing adequate medical care and with efficient administration (*Id.* § 23-17.5-2). Patients may associate and communicate privately with persons of their choice and shall be allowed freedom and privacy in sending and receiving mail (*Id.* § 23-17.5-12), and may manage their own financial affairs (*Id.* 23-17.5-15). If married, patients shall be assured of privacy for visits by their spouse; if both are inpatients in the facility, they may share a room unless medically contraindicated per written order of the physician and subject to the availability of accommodations within the facility (*Id.* § 23-17.5-16).

Mental health patients also have the rights to privacy and dignity under Rhode Island General Laws § 40.1-5-5, including, among others, the right to:

- Be provided with stationery, writing materials, and postage in reasonable amounts and to have free unrestricted, unopened, and uncensored use of the mails for letters.

- Be visited privately at all reasonable times by their personal physician, attorney, and clergy, and by other persons at all reasonable times unless the facility's administrator determines that a visitor or particular visitation time would not be in the best interests of patients and the administrator incorporates a statement for any denial of visiting rights in the individualized treatment record of the patient.

- Reasonable access to telephones to make and receive confidential calls unless good cause exists for denial of this right.

The developmentally disabled in community residences have the right to dignity, privacy, and humane care under § 40.1-22.1-5 and the right to be visited privately at all reasonable times by their personal physician, attorney, clergy, and the mental health advocate and to communicate by sealed mail or otherwise with persons of their choosing under § 40.1-24.5-5. Section 40.1-24.5-6 gives residents the right to have reasonable access to a telephone to make and receive confidential calls unless good cause exists for limiting this right.

South Carolina

The Bill of Rights for Residents of Long-Term Care Facilities specifies that each resident:

- May manage his or her personal finances unless the facility has been delegated in writing to carry out this responsibility.

- Must be treated with respect and dignity and assured of privacy during treatment and when receiving personal care.

- Must be allowed to associate and communicate privately with persons of his or her choice and be assured freedom and privacy in sending and receiving mail.

- Must be assured of privacy for visits of a conjugal nature.

- If married, be permitted to share a room with the spouse unless medically contraindicated (South Carolina Code § 44-81-40).

Except to the extent that the facility superintendent of an institution for the treatment of the mentally ill and mentally retarded determines the patient's medical needs require otherwise, each patient may:

- Communicate by sealed mail, by telephone, or otherwise with persons, including official agencies, inside or outside the institution.
- Receive visitors.
- Notwithstanding any limitations on the right of communication imposed by the superintendent, every patient may communicate with the Department of Mental Health, with the court which ordered his or her confinement, and with his or her counsel, legal guardian, personal physician, and clergy (*Id.* § 44-23-1030).

Mental health patients have the right to communicate by sealed mail, by telephone, or otherwise with persons including official agencies, inside or outside the institution. The institution must provide reasonable access to writing materials, stamps, and envelopes. They also have the right to receive visitors, including unrestricted visits by legal counsel, private physicians, or members of the clergy or an advocate of the South Carolina Protection and Advocacy System for the Handicapped, Inc., if such visits take place at reasonable hours, by appointment, or both. Each facility must have a designated area in which patients and visitors may speak privately, if desired.

South Dakota

Mentally ill patients have the right to a humane environment that affords appropriate individual privacy, individual dignity and reasonable protection from harm under § 27A-12-1, as do the mentally retarded under § 27B-8-1.

Tennessee

Nursing home patients in Tennessee have the minimum right, among others, to:

- Privacy during treatment and personal care. Residents/patients shall be assured of at least visual privacy in multibed rooms and in the bathtub, shower, and toilet rooms.
- If married, visit in private with their spouse, and, if not medically contraindicated and if space is available, have conjugal visits with their spouse and to share a room with their spouse.
- Visit in private with any person or persons during reasonable hours, subject to the right of the administrator to refuse access to the facility to any person if the presence of that person in the facility would be injurious to the health and safety of a resident or the staff, or would threaten the security of the property of the resident, staff, or facility.

- Communicate by telephone with any person they so choose.
- Delivery of their mail, unopened, on the business day it is received by the facility and to send mail to any person without interference by the facility.
- Manage financial affairs.
- Be treated with consideration, respect, and full recognition of their dignity and individuality.

Each facility shall respect a resident's right to the use and quiet enjoyment of his or her personal room or, in the case of multiple occupancy, that part of such resident's room designated for such resident's personal use. To this end, a resident shall have the right to close the room door unless the physician or registered nurse orders it to remain ajar or fully open. The staff of the facility shall have the right to check on a resident by coming to the door or into the room as needed to provide medical care, give personal care, or ensure the safety of the patient (Tennessee Code Annotated § 68-11-901).

Patients being treated for alcohol or drug use have the right to mail or other communications free from interception, reading, or censorship. The facility may adopt reasonable policies for the use of the telephone in the facility (*Id.* § 68-24-509).

Texas

Residents in personal care facilities have the right, among others, to:
- Manage their financial affairs.
- Send and receive unopened mail.
- Unaccompanied access to a telephone at a reasonable hour or in case of an emergency or personal crisis.
- Privacy.
- Unrestricted communication, including personal visitation with any person of the resident's choice, at any reasonable hour.
- A safe and decent living environment and considerate and respectful care that recognizes the dignity and individuality of the resident (Texas Health and Safety Code § 247.065).

Section 576.021 provides that patients receiving mental health services have the right to a humane treatment environment that provides reasonable protection from harm and appropriate privacy for personal needs.

Utah

The Health Facility Licensure Rules for nursing care facilities, Utah Administrative Code 434-150-4, specify that patients have the right, among others, to:

- Manage personal financial affairs.
- Be assured of confidential treatment of personal and medical records.
- Be treated with consideration, respect, and full recognition of dignity and individuality, including privacy in treatment and in care for personal needs.
- Associate with and communicate privately with persons of choice, and to send and receive personal mail unopened.
- If married, be assured of privacy for visits by their spouse and if both are patients in the facility, to be permitted to share a room.
- Be allowed privacy for visits with family, friends, clergy, social workers, or for professional or business purposes.
- Have reasonable access to telephones both to make and to receive confidential calls.

Patients in mental disease facilities have the rights to conduct private telephone conversations with family and friends *(Id.* R432-151-4).

Clients of mental retardation facilities have, among others, the right to:

- Manage their financial affairs.
- Have the opportunity for personal privacy and privacy during treatment and care of personal needs.
- Communicate, associate, and meet privately with individuals of their choice, including legal counsel and clergy, and to send and receive unopened mail.
- Have access to telephones with privacy for incoming and outgoing local and long distance calls except as contraindicated by factors identified within their individual program plans.
- If married, reside together as a couple when both reside in the facility *(Id.* R432-152-4).

Residents of residential care facilities have the privacy right *(Id.* R432-250-4) to:

- Be treated with respect, consideration, fairness, and full consideration of personal dignity and individuality.

- Privacy for visits with family, friends, clergy, social workers, ombudsmen, and advocacy representatives during reasonable hours.

- Privacy when receiving personal care or services.

- Share a room with a spouse, if both are residents.

- Send and receive mail unopened and have reasonable access to telephones both to make and to receive confidential calls.

- Manage and control personal cash resources.

Ambulatory surgical center patients have the right to privacy in treatment and care for personal needs (*Id.* R432-500-4), as do home health agency patients (*Id.* R432-700-3).

The Health Facility Licensure Rules for Specialty Hospital-Psychiatric, Utah Administrative Code R432-101-4, specifies that each patient shall be permitted to send and receive unopened mail, shall be afforded reasonable access to a telephone to make and receive unmonitored telephone calls, and shall be permitted to receive authorized visitors and speak to them in private.

Patients in mental health facilities have the right to communicate, by sealed mail or otherwise, with persons (including official agencies) inside or outside the facility and to receive visitors (Utah Code § 62A-12-245).

Vermont

The Vermont Bill of Rights for Hospital Patients specifies that a patient has the right to:

- Considerate and respectful care at all times and under all circumstances with recognition of his or her personal dignity.

- Every consideration of privacy concerning the patient's own medical care program. Case discussion, consultation, examination, and treatment are confidential. Those not directly involved in the patient's care must have the permission of the patient to be present. This right includes the right, upon request, to have a person of one's own sex present during certain parts of a physical examination, treatment, or procedure performed by a healthcare professional of the opposite sex, and the right not to remain disrobed any longer than is required for accomplishing the medical purpose for which the patient was asked to disrobe.

- Wear appropriate personal clothing and religious or other symbolic items so long as they do not interfere with diagnostic procedures or treatment (18 Vermont Statutes Annotated § 1852).

Virginia

Virginia hospitals must establish a protocol relating to the rights and responsibilities of patients that is based on the Joint Commission on Accreditation of Healthcare Organizations' standards (Virginia Code § 32.1-127).

Patients in nursing homes have, among others, the right to:

- Manage their own personal affairs or access to financial transactions made on their behalf if the facility has accepted written delegation of these financial affairs.

- Be treated with consideration, respect, and full recognition of their dignity and individuality, including privacy in treatment and care for personal needs.

- Associate with and communicate privately with persons of their choice and to send and receive personal mail unopened, unless medically contraindicated.

- If married, privacy for visits by their spouse and if both are inpatients, to share a room with their spouse unless medically contraindicated (*Id.* § 32.1-138).

Mentally ill patients have the right to send and receive sealed-letter mail under Virginia Code § 37.1-84.1.

Residents of adult care residences have the right, among others, to:

- Confidential treatment of their personal affairs and records.

- Respect for ordinary privacy in every aspect of daily living, including but not limited to the following:

  - In the care of personal needs except as assistance may be needed.

  - In any medical examination or health-related consultations the resident may have at the residence.

  - In communications, in writing or by telephone.

  - During visitations by other persons.

  - In the resident's room or portion thereof. Residents shall be permitted to have guests or other residents in their rooms unless to do so would infringe upon the rights of other residents. Staff may not enter residents' room without making their presence known except in an emergency or in accordance with safety oversight requirements included in regulations of the State Board of Social Services.

- In visits with the resident's spouse. If both are residents of
the residence, they are permitted, but not required, to share a
room unless otherwise provided in their resident's agreements
(*Id.* § 63.1-182.1).

Washington

Under Revised Code of Washington § 74.42.050, residents of nursing
homes shall be treated with consideration, respect, and full recognition of
their dignity and individuality. Residents shall be allowed to communicate,
associate, meet privately with individuals of their choice, and participate in
social, religious, and community group activities unless this infringes on
the rights of other residents (*Id.* § 74.42.110).

Under Revised Code of Washington § 71.12.570, no person in a private establishment for the treatment of mental illness shall be restrained
from sending written communications of the fact of his or her detention in
such establishment to a friend, relative, or other person. The physician in
charge of such person and the person in charge of such establishment shall
send each such communication to the person to whom it is addressed. A
resident also has the same essential rights as just detailed for nursing home
residents.

West Virginia

Patients in nursing home and residential care facilities have, as a minimum,
patients' rights as prescribed under federal law.

Wisconsin

Wisconsin's Medical Assistance Laws, Wisconsin Statutes § 49.498, Requirements for Skilled Nursing Facilities, specifies that residents have the
right, among others, to:

- Privacy with regard to accommodations, medical treatment, written and telephonic communications, visits, and meetings of family
and resident groups, except that this statute does not require the
provision of a private room.
- Confidentiality of personal records.

This statute also requires the facility to permit immediate access to
the resident by various state and federal officials, immediate family, and
those who provide legal, social, health, or other services to the resident.
Facilities may not require residents to deposit personal funds with the nursing facility (*Id.*).

Wisconsin Statutes § 50.09 details rights of residents in nursing homes and community-based residential facilities. Among them are the right to:

- Private and unrestricted communications with the residents' family, physician, attorney, and any other person, unless medically contraindicated, except that communications with public officials or with the residents' attorney shall not be restricted in any event. The right to private and unrestricted communications includes, but is not limited, to:

  - Receiving, sending, and mailing sealed, unopened correspondence. No resident's incoming or outgoing correspondence shall be opened, delayed, held, or censored.

  - Reasonable access to a telephone for private communications.

  - Opportunity for private visits.

- Manage their own financial affairs unless the residents delegate such responsibility to the facility and the facility accepts it.

- Treatment with courtesy, respect, and full recognition of residents' dignity and individuality.

- Privacy in treatment, living arrangements, and in caring for personal needs, including, but not limited to:

  - Privacy for visits by spouses. If both spouses are residents of the same facility, the facility shall permit them to share a room unless medically contraindicated.

  - Privacy concerning health care. Case discussion, consultation, examination, and treatment are confidential and shall be conducted discreetly. Persons not directly involved in residents' care require the residents' permission to be present at such times.

  - Confidentiality in health and personal records.

Wisconsin's State Alcohol, Drug Abuse, Developmental Disabilities, and Mental Health Act also specifies rights for such patients, including the right to a humane psychological and physical environment within the hospital facilities that shall be designed to afford comfort and safety, to promote dignity, and to ensure privacy (*Id.* § 51.61). This statute adds that patients have a right not to be filmed or taped unless patients sign an informed and voluntary consent that specifically authorizes a named individual or group to film or tape patients for a particular purpose or project during a specified time period. Patients may also see visitors and make and receive telephone calls within reasonable limits. Finally, this law requires the hospital to ensure that patients have reasonable privacy protection in such matters as toileting and bathing.

Wyoming

The Wyoming Patient Bill of Rights for the State Hospital promulgated by the Board of Charities and Reform includes the right to:

- Treatment and related services in a setting and under conditions that are most supportive of the patient's personal liberty and restrict such liberty only to the extent necessarily consistent with the person's treatment needs, applicable requirements of law, and applicable judicial orders.

- A humane treatment environment that affords a patient reasonable protection from harm and appropriate privacy for personal needs.

- Protection of personal privacy and dignity.

- If admitted on a residential or inpatient care basis:

  - Converse with others privately.

  - Have convenient and reasonable access to the telephone.

  - Send and receive uncensored and unopened mail.

Conclusion

Every jurisdiction provides for the privacy rights of patients. Among the most important are the right to privacy in treatment and in personal care, the right to private communications and visits, and the right to manage personal and financial affairs. Chapter 3 discusses another important aspect of patients' rights to privacy—the confidentiality of medical information.

3

Privacy and Confidentiality of Medical Information

Introduction

Every state and the federal government provide for confidentiality of medical records and medical information. And, as discussed in Chapter 1, even if the law did not protect patient information, medical ethics does. Both the Hippocratic Oath and the American Medical Association's Principles of Medical Ethics require physicians to safeguard patient confidences. In addition, the Joint Commission's *1994 Accreditation Manual for Hospitals* specifies in Standard IM.2.1 that the facility must determine the need for and appropriate levels of confidentiality of healthcare information. IM.2.3 adds that the facility has a mechanism to safeguard medical records/information against unauthorized access or use. Aside from these industry standards, the physician-patient and similar privileges and federal and state laws provide for the confidentiality of medical information.

The Physician-Patient Privilege

Most states have statutes that prohibit physicians from disclosing information that they learned as a result of treating patients. The purpose of this privilege is to encourage patients to disclose everything relevant to their conditions to their physicians in a full and frank manner so that physicians may treat them properly. The privilege means that patients have a privilege to refuse to disclose and to prevent doctors from disclosing information they told their doctors in confidence during treatment. The privilege usually covers not only oral information, but also any information the physician obtains during the course of examination or treatment, such as test results, diagnoses, and medical advice. Incidental information, such as the patient's occupation, address, and age, is usually not privileged. The practical effect of this privilege is that a physician cannot disclose confidential information learned during medical examination or treatments in court unless the patient waives the privilege. The privilege may not apply to criminal trials.

The privilege is the patient's, not the physician's. If the patient waives the privilege, the physician cannot invoke it and the court may compel the physician to waive it. If the patient is deceased or incompetent, the personal representative or guardian, respectively, may assert the privilege on the patient's behalf. Statutes or court decisions typically provide that a patient waives the privilege by filing a malpractice action so that the doctor may use information gained during treatment to defend himself or herself. The law may make this privilege inapplicable in certain circumstances, such as child or elder abuse reporting, communicable disease reporting, and illegal attempts by the patient to obtain drugs.

Besides physician-patient privileges, some jurisdictions recognize other privileges, such as psychologist or psychiatrist privileges. In addition, other health professionals, such as nurses, may be covered by physician-patient and similar privileges so that they cannot divulge information obtained while assisting the physician or other licensed professional.

Because these privileges are complex, a provider should see a healthcare attorney before disclosing any information gained from a patient during the course of treatment.

Federal Confidentiality Laws

The Condition of Participation: Medical Records Services of the Health Care Financing Administration specifies that hospitals must have a procedure for ensuring the confidentiality of patient records to qualify for Medicare funds. The facility may release information forms or copies of records only to authorized individuals, and the hospital must ensure that unauthorized individuals cannot gain access to or alter patient records. The hospital must release medical records only in accordance with federal or state laws, court orders, or subpoenas (42 CFR, Chapter 4, § 482.24).

State Laws

Alabama

Records and information regarding patients are confidential, with access to them determined by the governing board of the facility [Alabama Administrative Code r. 420-5-7.07 (h) (Rules of the Alabama State Board of Health Division of Licensure and Certification)]. These rules permit inspectors for licensure or surveyors for membership in professional organizations to review medical records as necessary to determine compliance with licensure or membership requirements.

Records and information regarding patients in nursing homes are also confidential under these rules. Access is limited to designated staff members, physicians, and others having professional responsibility and to members of the state board of health (*Id.* r. 420-5-10-.16).

Alabama provides for confidentiality of information concerning Medicaid recipients in Alabama Code § 22-6-9, as well as the right to privacy of long-term residential healthcare patients who file complaints with the ombudsmen (*Id.* § 22-5A-6).

Alaska

Alaska's Constitution sets forth the right to privacy. In *Gunnerud v. State*, 611 P.2d 69 (Alaska, 1980), the court held that it would be an unwarranted infringement of a witness's privacy to grant access to his or her private medical records unless the material was relevant.

Patients have the right to confidentiality for their medical records and treatments according to Alaska Administrative Code Title 7 § 12.890 (a) (7). Information regarding a patient may be released without consent only to:

- A person authorized by court order.
- Healthcare providers if a medical emergency arises.
- Research projects authorized by the governing board, if provision is made to preserve anonymity in the reported results.
- Other persons, such as those to whom disclosure of child abuse is required by law *(Id.* § 13.130; Alaska Statutes §§ 47.17.010 through 47.17.070).

A facility may also release records and information regarding a patient to the patient or to an individual for whom the patient, or legally designated representative of the patient, has given written consent to disclosure (*Id.* § 18.23.065).

Arizona

Arizona Healthcare Institutions Licensure Regulations provide that medical record information may be released only with the written consent of the patient or legal guardian, or in accordance with law, and that in hospitals that have designated psychiatric or substance abuse units, confidentiality of medical records must be maintained as required by Arizona law (Arizona Revised Statutes § 36-509; Arizona Compilation Administrative Rules & Regulations, 9-10-221).

Several other Arizona statutes also provide for confidentiality, including the following protections:

- The board of medical examiners must maintain confidentiality of patient records and the like and must not release such records to the public (Arizona Revised Statutes § 32-1451.01).
- Nursing care institutions must assure patients of confidential handling of personal and medical records and may release such records only after written consent of the patient or responsible party, except as otherwise required or permitted by law (*Id.* § 36-447.17).

Arkansas

Because medical records are confidential, only personnel authorized by the administrator shall have access to them. Written consent of the patient is necessary for authority to release medical records [Arkansas Register 0601

U (Medical Records)]. Medical records may not be removed from the hospital except upon issuance of a subpoena by a court that has authority to issue such a subpoena [*Id*. 0601 (V) and 0601(W)].

Adult care homes must ensure that residents have medical and financial records kept in confidence (*Id.* § 36-448.08).

California

California's Confidentiality of Medical Information Act, California Civil Code § 56.10, confirms patients' rights to privacy in their medical records by governing the release of patient-identifiable information by healthcare providers. The Health and Safety Code § 1795.12 provides for patient or patient representative access upon request and payment of reasonable clerical costs. Violation of this section may result in disciplinary action by the licensing authority. California Civil Code § 56.10(c) also provides for permissive access by the following entities:

- Healthcare providers.
- Insurers to the extent necessary to obtain payment.
- Credentialing committees.
- Licensing or accrediting bodies (however, the facility may not permit the licensing or accrediting body to remove patient identifiable information unless expressly permitted or required by law).
- County coroner.
- Researchers.
- Employers, if the medical treatment was at the prior request and payment of the employer [*Id*. § 56.10(a)].

The code also provides for mandatory disclosure to authorized representatives of patients when the patient has executed a valid release. Violations of this statute constitute a misdemeanor if the unauthorized release harms the patient (*Id*. § 1798.57). In addition, the patient may recover actual damages, punitive damages not to exceed $3,000, and attorney's fees not to exceed $1,000 (*Id*. § 56.35).

Recipients of medical information under California Civil Code section 56.10 may not further disclose it without a new authorization (*Id*. § 56.13). But unless a patient specifically requests in writing to the contrary, a provider may release at its discretion any of the following information, upon an inquiry concerning a specific patient:

- Patient's name, address, age, and sex.

- General description of the reason for treatment (whether an injury, a burn, poisoning, or some unrelated condition).

- General nature of the injury, burn, poisoning, or other condition.

- General condition of the patient.

- Any information that is not medical information [*Id.* § 56.05(c)].

California Code of Regulations Title 22, § 70707(b)(8), provides that anyone not directly connected with a patient's care must obtain written permission of the patient before any provider may make medical records available.

Regulations specify that in addition to general acute hospitals, the following other types of facilities must maintain confidentiality of patient records:

- Acute psychiatric hospitals [*Id.* § 71551(a)].

- Skilled nursing facilities [*Id.* § 72543(b)].

- Intermediate care facilities [*Id.* § 73543(b)].

- Home health agencies [*Id.* § 74731(c)].

- Primary care clinics [*Id.* § 75055(b)].

- Psychology clinics [*Id.* § 75343(b)].

- Psychiatric health facilities [*Id.* § 77143(a)].

- Adult day health facilities [*Id.* § 78433].

- Chemical dependency recovery hospitals [*Id.* § 79347(b)].

Colorado

Colorado Revised Statutes § 25-1-120 specifies that among the rights of patients of nursing and intermediate care facilities is the right to have privacy in treatment, including confidentiality in the handling of personal and medical records.

Section 18-4-412 makes it a felony to knowingly obtain, steal, disclose to an unauthorized person, or copy a medical record or medical information without proper authorization. The statute defines *proper authorization* as a written authorization signed by the patient or his duly designated representative or an appropriate order of court or authorized possession pursuant to law or regulation for claims processing, possession for medical audit or quality assurance purposes, possession by a consulting physician to the patient, or possession by hospital personnel for record-keeping and billing purposes.

Connecticut

Connecticut General Statute 19a-550, titled, "Patient's Bill of Rights," provides for patients' rights to confidentiality generally. Section 19a-550 provides that a nursing home or chronic disease hospital must assure any patient of the confidential treatment of his or her personal and medical records and may approve or refuse their release to any individual outside the facility, except in case of the patient's transfer to another healthcare institution or as required by law or third-party payment contract.

Delaware

Delaware Code Annotated Title 16, § 1121(6), governing the rights of patients in sanatoria, rest homes, nursing homes, boarding homes, and related institutions, specifies that such facilities shall treat personal and medical records confidentially and not make them public without the consent of the patient or resident.

District of Columbia

D.C. Code § 32-255(a) governs the confidentiality of medical records and information at D.C. General Hospital. It provides that medical records and other information and/or materials pertaining to any patient shall not be disclosed for any reason other than the medical care of the patient without the informed written consent of the patient or his or her legally authorized representative. Each request must be specific; blanket consent may not be secured.

Florida

Florida Administrative Code Annotated rule 10D-28.110(10)(f)(5) provides that a hospital facility may not release clinical record information without the written consent of the patient, family, or other legally responsible party. Rule 10D-28.110(10)(f)(4) directs hospitals to protect the confidentiality of clinical information and communication between staff and patients.

Rule 10D-28.158(3) provides that hospital patient records shall have a privileged and confidential status and shall not be disclosed without the consent of the person to whom they pertain, but appropriate disclosure may be made without such consent to:

- Hospital personnel for use in connection with the treatment of the patient.
- Hospital personnel only for internal hospital administrative purposes associated with the treatment.

- The Hospital Cost Containment Board.

Rule 10D-29.082(2) provides that nursing home clinical records are confidential and may not be released without written permission of the patient or guardian, except to persons or agencies with a legitimate professional need or regulatory authority. Similarly, § 21G-17.001(1) provides that dental records are confidential and may not be released unless authorized by the patient in writing.

Georgia

No physician, hospital, or healthcare facility shall be required to release any medical information concerning a patient except to the Department of Human Resources and its subelements, unless the patient, his or her parents, or guardian authorize such release in writing; the patient waives any privilege; a law, statute, or regulation requires release; a court orders release; or the records are subpoenaed. Georgia Code Annotated § 24-9-40 (Michie 1991). This section does not apply to psychiatrists or to hospitals in which the patient is or has been treated solely for mental illness.

Data concerning the diagnosis, treatment, or health of anyone enrolled in an HMO is confidential and may not be disclosed except upon consent of the enrollee or pursuant to statute or court order or in the event of a claim or litigation between the enrollee and the HMO (*Id.* § 33-21-23).

Hawaii

Hawaii's retention of medical records statute requires medical records to be retained "in a manner that will preserve the confidentiality of the information in the record" (Hawaii Revised Statutes § 622-58).

Idaho

Idaho Code § 54-1814 lists failure to safeguard the confidentiality of medical records or other medical information pertaining to identifiable patients as a ground for medical discipline.

Section 39-1310 makes confidential all information received by the licensing agency that would identify individual residents or patients.

Illinois

Every patient has the right to confidentiality in healthcare information under 410 Illinois Compiled Statutes 50/3. Healthcare providers may not disclose the nature or details of services provided to patients without written consent from the patient or the patient's guardian. And, where two or more patient confidentiality statutes conflict, the more stringent applies (735 ILCS 5/8-2002).

Nursing home residents' rights have additional protection under 210 ILCS 45/2-206. The health department must respect the confidentiality of resident records and may not divulge or disclose the contents of a record in any manner that identifies a resident, except upon a resident's death, to a relative or guardian, or under judicial proceedings. No one may make confidential medical, social, personal, or financial information identifying a resident available for public inspection in a manner that identifies a resident.

Indiana

Indiana Code § 16-4-8-8 provides that the original health record of the patient is the property of the provider and thus may be used by the provider without specific written authorization for legitimate business purposes. However, the provider shall at all times protect the confidentiality of the record and may only disclose the identity of the patient when it is essential to the provider's business use, to quality assurance, or to peer review.

Iowa

Iowa Code § 22.7 makes certain public records confidential, including hospital records, medical records, and professional counselor records of the condition, diagnosis, care, or treatment of a patient or former patient or a counselee or former counselee, including outpatients.

Section 514B.30 prohibits officers, directors, trustees, partners, and employees of HMOs from testifying to or making public disclosure of privileged communications and may not release the names of its membership list of enrollees.

Iowa Administrative Code rule 441-81.13(5) specifies that residents of nursing facilities have the right to personal privacy and confidentiality of personal and clinical records.

Rule 481-57.49(135C) specifies that residents of residential care facilities have a right to confidential treatment of all information contained in their medical, personal, and financial records, as do rule 481-59.49(135C) for skilled nursing facilities and rule 481-58.44(135C) for intermediate care facilities.

Kansas

Kansas Administrative Regulations § 28-34-9a(d)(5) specifies that records shall be confidential. Only persons authorized by the hospital governing body, including individuals designated by the licensing agency to verify compliance with statutes or regulations and for disease control investigations, shall have access to the records.

Kentucky

902 Kentucky Administrative Regulation 20:016 § 3(11)(c) states that only authorized personnel shall be permitted access to patient records. Patient information shall be released only on authorization of the patient, the patient's guardian, or the executor of his or her estate.

Louisiana

Nursing Home Residents' Bill of Rights, § 2010.8, provides that all residents have the right to have confidentiality in the treatment of personal and medical records [*Id.* § 40:2010.8(A)(8)].

Patients of professional corporations have a right to confidentiality (*Id.* §§ 12:905 and 12:906). Shareholders of such corporations shall not have access to any records or communications pertaining to medical services rendered by, or any other affairs of, the corporation, except as provided by section 12:913B.

Professional veterinary medicine corporations (*Id.* §§ 12:1155 and 12:1156), professional psychology corporations (§§ 12:1134 and 12:1135), professional dental corporations (§§ 12:985 and 12:986), and professional optometry corporations (§§ 12:1115 and 12:1116) have similar requirements.

Maine

The Regulations for the Licensure of General and Specialty Hospitals in the State of Maine states that only authorized personnel may have access to patient records, that written consent of the patient must be presented as authority for the release of medical information, and that medical records generally cannot be removed from the hospital except upon subpoena (State of Maine, Regulations for the Licensure of General and Specialty Hospitals, chapter XII, § A).

Maryland

Maryland Health-General Code Annotated § 4-302 provides for confidentiality of medical records. Healthcare providers shall keep the medical record confidential and disclose it only as provided by law. However, this statute does not apply to information:

- Not kept in the medical record of a patient or recipient that is related to the administration of the facility, including the following:

  - Risk management.

  - Quality assurance.

  - Any activities of medical or dental review committees that are confidential.

- Governed by the federal confidentiality of alcohol and drug abuse patient regulations.

- Governed by the developmental disability confidentiality provisions.

Code of Maryland Regulations Title 10, § 07.10.12 requires home health agencies to have proper safeguards for clinical record information against illegal or unauthorized use. Regulations for HMOs have more detailed requirements, which state that all information contained in the medical records and information received from physicians, surgeons, or hospitals, incident to the doctor-patient or hospital-patient relationship shall be kept confidential and may not be disclosed without the consent of the patient, except for research or education or the Department of Health and Mental Hygiene's review [*Id.* Title 10, § 07.11.05(B)].

Massachusetts

Massachusetts General Laws Chapter 214, § 1B, gives a person a right against unreasonable, substantial, or serious interference with his or her privacy and may sue for a violation thereof. In *Tower v. Hirschhorn*, 397 Mass. 581, 492 N.E. 2d 728 (1986), the court found that a physician's disclosure of confidential medical information to two people without the patient's consent was sufficient to find an invasion of privacy under this law.

Every patient or resident of a hospital, institution for the care of unwed mothers, clinic, infirmary, convalescent or nursing home, or home for the aged has the right to confidentiality of all records and communications (Massachusetts General Laws chapter 111, § 70E). This section does not prevent any third-party reimburser from inspecting and copying, in the ordinary course of determining eligibility for or entitlement to benefits, records relating to diagnosis, treatment, or other services provided to any person for which coverage, benefit, or reimbursement is claimed so long as the policy provides for such access or in connection with any peer or utilization review. Confidential information in medical records may only be provided upon written authority of the patient or the executor of his or her estate (*Id.*)

Michigan

Under Michigan Compiled Laws § 333.20201, patients of health facilities and agencies are entitled to confidential treatment of personal and medical records and may refuse their release to a person outside the facility except as required because of transfer to another healthcare facility or as required by law or third-party payment contract. Otherwise, a third party shall not be given a copy of a patient's or a resident's medical record without prior authorization of the patient or resident.

Minnesota

Minnesota Statutes § 144.651(16) assures patients and residents of healthcare facilities of confidential treatment of their personal and medical records. Patients and residents may approve or refuse their release to any individual outside the facility. The facility shall notify residents when any individual outside the facility requests personal records and may select someone to accompany them when the records or information is the subject of a personal interview.

Mississippi

According to Mississippi Code § 41-9-67, hospital records are not public records, and patients have a privilege of confidence in them.

Under section 41-83-17, private review agents may not disclose or publish individual medical records or other confidential medical information obtained in the performance of utilization review activities without the patient's authorization or a court order.

Missouri

Missouri Revised Statutes § 198.032 provides for confidentiality of reports of complaints and records, including medical, social, personal, or financial records, of residents of convalescent, nursing, and boarding homes held by the Missouri Department of Social Services. Rights of residents of such facilities include the right to be ensured confidential treatment of all information contained in their records, which encompasses data contained in an automatic data bank [*Id.* § 198.088(1)(6)(n)]. Section 192.067 requires the Department of Health to maintain the confidentiality of medical record information abstracted by or reported to the Department of Health.

Missouri Code Regulations Title 13, 50-20.021(d)(7), notes that hospitals cannot release medical records or information without the written consent of the patient or his or her legal representative.

Montana

Montana's constitution contains a right to privacy (Montana Constitution article II, § 10). Of course, the doctor-patient privilege, Montana Code § 26-1-805, protects the patient's confidentiality. Further, § 50-16-529, which specifies conditions under which patients' healthcare information may be disclosed without their authorization based on need to know, contains provisions requiring the recipient to treat the information as confidential.

Montana puts teeth into confidentiality requirements by making it a crime to willfully misrepresent one's identity or purpose (false pretenses) or to use bribery or theft to examine healthcare information (*Id.* § 50-16-551).

The *Montana Hospital Association Manual*, Chapters 23 and 24, speaks of maintaining records to protect their secrecy.

Nebraska

Revised Statutes of Nebraska §§ 44-32,171 and 44-4725 note that data or information pertaining to the diagnosis, treatment, or health of any enrollee or applicant of an HMO is confidential.

Section 68-1025 makes confidential information regarding applicants for or recipients of medical assistance.

Nevada

Nevada Revised Statutes § 449.720 specifies that all patients of medical facilities have the right to retain their privacy concerning their programs of medical care, including confidentiality of all communications and records concerning them.

New Hampshire

New Hampshire's general confidentiality statute is New Hampshire Revised Statutes Annotated § 151:13, which provides that information other than reports relating to vital statistics received by the Department of Health and Human Services, Division of Public Health Services, through inspection or otherwise, are confidential and shall not be disclosed publicly except in a proceeding involving the question of licensure or revocation of license. The Hospital and Sanitaria Patients' Bill of Rights specifies that the patient shall be assured of confidential treatment of all information contained in his or her personal and clinical record, including that stored in an automatic data bank, and his or her written consent shall be required for the release of information to anyone not otherwise authorized by law to receive it (*Id.* § 151:21).

Records of residents of sheltered care facilities are also confidential [New Hampshire Code Administrative Rules Hospital Department of Health & Human Services Regulations (General Hospitals) He-P 804.04(c)]. Clinical records of outpatient clinics, residential treatment and rehabilitation facilities, and home healthcare providers shall be safeguarded against unauthorized record use (*Id.* He-P 806.10, 807.07, and 809.07). Clinical laboratories must keep records and reports of tests confidential [*Id.* He-P 808.12(e)].

New Hampshire Revised Statutes Annotated § 318-B:12 makes healthcare practitioners responsible for keeping separate records of receipt and disposition of controlled drugs, "so as not to breach the confidentiality of patient records."

New Jersey

Facilities must develop procedures to protect medical records from unauthorized use [New Jersey Administrative Code Title 8, § 8:43B-7.4 (Supp. 1989), Standards for Hospital Facilities].

New Mexico

Section 14-6-1 states that all health information that identifies specific individuals as patients is strictly confidential and is not a matter of public record or accessible to the public even though it is in the custody of a governmental agent or a licensed health facility. The custodian of such information may furnish it upon request "to a governmental agency or its agent, a state educational institution, a duly organized state or county association of licensed physicians or dentists, a licensed health facility, or staff committees of such facilities." Statistical studies and research reports may be published if they do not identify individual patients or otherwise violate the physician-patient privilege.

According to the New Mexico Hospital Association Legal Handbook, chapter 5B (rev. 1981), all hospitals should treat all patient information as confidential and should not divulge it to anyone other than the patient's physician without the patient's written consent. The hospital should notify the patient of any subpoena it receives concerning his or her records in any case in which the patient is not a party and should not release the records unless the patient consents or the facility receives a court order. The handbook notes that unauthorized release of information from the patient's medical record may give rise to civil liability.

New York

New York Public Health Law § 2803-c (McKinney, 1992), Rights of Patients in Certain Medical Facilities, provides that every patient shall have the right to confidentiality in the treatment of personal and medical records. New York Social Services Law § 461-d (McKinney, 1992) has a similar requirement with regard to residents in adult care facilities.

New York Compilation of Codes, Rules & Regulations Title 10, § 405.10(a)(5) of the Department of Health, Health Facilities Series H-40, notes that hospitals shall ensure the confidentiality of patient records. Section 405.7, titled "Patients' Rights," specifies that one patient right is to confidentiality of all information and records pertaining to his or her treatment, except as otherwise provided by law.

North Carolina

North Carolina's physician-patient communications privilege statute states that confidential information in medical records shall be furnished only on the authorization of the patient or, if deceased, his or her executor, administrator, or next of kin or if ordered by a judge (North Carolina General Statute § 8-53).

Medical information concerning enrollees or applicants in HMOs is confidential (*Id.* § 58-67-180).

North Dakota

North Dakota's Administrative Code § 33-07-01-16(a) through (c), Hospital Licensing Rules, requires hospitals to keep medical records confidential. Only authorized persons shall have access to the record, and written consent of the patient must be presented as authority for the release of medical information. Medical records generally shall not be removed from the hospital environment except upon subpoena. Section 33-07-03-13-4 specifies that all information contained in clinical records of long-term care facilities shall be treated as confidential and may be disclosed only to authorized persons.

Ohio

Medical records of persons covered by HMOs are confidential and shall not be released without the written consent of the covered person or a responsible party (*Id.*).

Section 3727.14 prohibits disclosing the name or social security number of a patient or physician in data, except that § 3727.11 requires hospitals to furnish such numbers to the Department of Health.

Oklahoma

Oklahoma Statutes Title 43A, § 1-109, makes medical records both confidential and privileged. Such information is available only to persons or agencies actively engaged in patient treatment or related administrative work. No such information shall be released to anyone not involved in treatment without a written release by the patient or, if the patient is a minor or if a guardian has been appointed, the guardian of the patient, or a court order [*Id.* Title 43A, § 1-109(A)(l)]. Oklahoma statutes make it unprofessional conduct for a medical professional to willfully betray a professional secret to the detriment of the patient (*Id.* Title 59, § 509).

Nursing homes, rest homes, specialized homes, and group homes for the developmentally disabled or physically handicapped must ensure that every resident receives respect and privacy in his or her medical care program. Case discussion, consultation, examination, and treatment shall remain confidential and personal, and medical records shall be confidential (*Id.* Title 63, § 1-1918 and § 1-818.20).

Oregon

Oregon Administrative Rules 333-70-055(18) require medical record departments to maintain written policies on the release of medical record information, including patient access to medical records.

Oregon Administrative Rules § 333-505-050(12) requires healthcare providers to take precautions to protect confidentiality of patient medical records. Further, Oregon Revised Statutes § 192.525 declares that the policy of the State of Oregon requires public and private healthcare providers to protect patients' rights of confidentiality of their medical records. Each provider must develop guidelines to ensure this protection (*Id.* § 192.530).

Persons other than the patient who have received access to a patient's records may not disclose the contents to anyone without permission or as otherwise provided by law [*Id.* § 179.505(12)].

Pennsylvania

28 Pennsylvania Code § 115.27 requires hospitals to treat all medical records as confidential. Only authorized personnel shall have access to the records. The written authorization of the patient shall be presented and then maintained in the original record as authority for release of medical infor-

mation outside the hospital. However, 42 Pennsylvania Consolidated Statutes § 6155 gives any patient whose medical charts or records are subpoenaed, any person acting on his or her behalf, and the healthcare facility having custody of the charts or records standing to apply to the court for a protective order denying, restricting, or otherwise limiting access to and use of the copies or records. Under 49 Pennsylvania Code § 16.61, revealing personally identifiable facts that were obtained as a result of the physician-patient relationship, without the prior consent of the patient, except as authorized or required by statute, is unprofessional conduct.

Patients of ambulatory surgical facilities have the right under 28 Pennsylvania Code § 553.12 to have records pertaining to their medical care treated as confidential, except as otherwise provided by law or third-party contractual arrangements.

Section 117.41(6)(8) requires emergency services to have the same policies on confidentiality of emergency room records as those that apply to other hospital medical records. The identity and general condition of the patient may be released to the public after the next of kin have been notified.

Ambulatory surgical facilities must also treat records as confidential, and only authorized personnel shall have access (*Id.* § 563.9).

Long-term care nursing facilities must ensure the confidentiality of medical records. Patients may approve or refuse the release of their personal and medical records to an individual outside the facility, except in case of a transfer to another healthcare institution or as required by statute or third-party payment contract (*Id.* § 201.29). Subscribers of HMOs have the right to have all records pertaining to the subscriber's medical care treated as confidential unless disclosure is necessary to interpret the application of their contract to their care or unless disclosure is otherwise provided for by law [*Id.* § 9.77(a)(8)].

Rhode Island

Rhode Island General Laws § 5-37.3-3-2 (9)(2), the Confidentiality of Health Care Information Act, established "safeguards for maintaining the integrity of confidential health care information that relates to an individual." Section 5-37.3-3(c) defines "confidential health care information" as "all information relating to a patient's health care history, diagnosis, condition, treatment, or evaluation obtained from a health care provider who has treated the patient." The statute requires that except as otherwise specifically provided by law, a patient's confidential healthcare information may not be released without the patient's consent or the consent of an authorized representative, except:

- To a physician, dentist, or other medical personnel who believe in good faith that the information is necessary to diagnose or treat the individual in a medical or dental emergency.

- To medical peer review committees or the State Board of Medical Review.

- To law enforcement personnel if someone is in danger from the patient, if the patient tries to get narcotics from the healthcare provider illegally, in child abuse cases, and in gunshot wound cases.

- For coordinating healthcare services and to educate and train within the same healthcare facility.

- To insurers to adjudicate health insurance claims.

- To malpractice insurance carriers or lawyers if the healthcare provider anticipates a medical liability action.

- To a court or lawyer or medical liability insurance carrier if a patient brings a medical liability action against the provider.

- To public health authorities in order to carry out their functions.

- To the state medical examiner in the event of a fatality that comes under his or her jurisdiction.

- Concerning information directly related to a claim for workers' compensation.

- To the attorneys for a healthcare provider when release is necessary to receive adequate legal representation.

- To school authorities of disease, health screening, and/or immunization information required by the school or when a school-age child transfers from one school or school district to another.

- To a law enforcement agency to protect the legal interests of an insurance institution agent or insurance-support organization in preventing and prosecuting the perpetration of fraud.

- To a grand jury or court pursuant to a subpoena when the information is required for the investigation or prosecution of criminal wrongdoing by a healthcare provider and the information is unavailable from any other source.

- To the state board of elections pursuant to a subpoena when required to determine the eligibility of a person to vote by mail due to illness or disability.

- To certify the nature of permanency of a person's illness or disability, the date when the patient was last examined, and that it would be an undue hardship for the person to vote at the polls so he or she may obtain a mail ballot.

- To the central cancer registry.
- To the Medicaid fraud control unit of the attorney general's office for the investigation or prosecution of criminal or civil wrongdoing by a healthcare provider in connection with provision of medical care to Medicaid recipients. However, any information so obtained may not be used in any criminal proceeding against the patient on whom the information is obtained [*Id.* § 5-37.3-4(b)].

A hospital may release the fact of a patient's admission and a general description of his or her condition to his or her relatives, friends, and the news media.

The statute also provides that third parties receiving a patient's confidential healthcare information must establish security procedures, including limiting access to those who have a "need to know"; identifying those who have responsibility for maintaining security procedures for such information; providing a written statement to each employee about the necessity of maintaining the confidentiality of the information and the penalties for unauthorized disclosure; and not taking disciplinary action against anyone who reports a violation of these rules [*Id.* § 5-37.3-5(c)].

South Carolina

The South Carolina Department for Health and Environmental Control Regulation for Minimum Standards for Licensing of Hospitals and Institutional General Infirmaries states that medical records will be treated as confidential (South Carolina Code of Regulations 61-16, § 601.7).

The Bill of Rights for Residents of Long-Term Care facilities provides for confidential treatment of personal and medical records. It specifies that residents may approve or disapprove release of their personal and medical records to any individual outside the facility, except they may not refuse in the case of transfer to another healthcare institution or when disclosure is required by law or third-party payment contract (*Id.* § 44-81-40).

Section 38-33-260 makes health records in the custody of HMOs confidential.

South Dakota

Administrative Rules of South Dakota 44:04:09:04 states that hospitals and nursing homes must have written policies and procedures pertaining to the confidentiality and safeguarding of medical records.

Tennessee

Tennessee Code Annotated § 68-11-304 specifies that hospital records, except as otherwise provided by law, are not public records, and nothing in the medical records statutes should be considered to impair any privilege of confidentiality conferred by law on patients, their personal representatives, or their heirs.

The law concerning the rights of nursing home residents and patients states that every nursing home resident has the right to have his or her records kept confidential and private (*Id.* § 68-11-901).

Texas

Texas Department of Health, Hospital Licensing Standard chapter 12 § 8.7.3.1, covering special care facilities, states that such facility shall protect medical records against loss, damage, destruction, and unauthorized use by safeguarding the confidentiality of medical record information and allowing access and/or release only under court order; by written authorization of the resident unless the physician has documented in the record to do so would be harmful to the physical, mental, or emotional health of the resident; as allowed by state licensing agency law and rules for licensure inspection purposes and reporting of communicable disease information; or as specifically allowed by federal or state laws relating to facilities caring for residents with AIDS or related disorders.

Under Texas Insurance Code article 20A.17(c)(2) (West, 1992), medical, hospital, and health records of enrollees and records of physicians and providers providing service under independent contract with an HMO are subject only to such examination as is necessary for an ongoing quality of health assurance program concerning healthcare procedures and outcome in accordance with an approved plan. The plan shall provide for adequate protection of confidentiality of medical information.

Utah

All hospital medical records must be kept confidential. Only authorized personnel may have access to medical records. The patient or his or her legal representative must give written consent to release medical information to unauthorized persons (Utah Administrative Rules 432-100-7.404). Rule 432-100-7.414 requires hospitals to have written policies approved by the medical staff relating to release of information, including child abuse records, psychiatric records, and drug and alcohol abuse records, and for confidentiality of medical records.

Utah Code Annotated § 26-25-1(3) allows healthcare providers to release confidential information only to state agencies, such as the Department of Human Services or the Utah State Medical Association for efficiency, quality control, and research purposes. Section 26-25-2 places restrictions on the use of such data to ensure confidentiality. Section 26-25-3 provides that all information, including information required for the medical and health section of birth certificates, interviews, reports, statements, memoranda, or other data provided under the health code, and any findings or conclusions resulting from medical studies are privileged communications. Section 26-25-4 adds that all such information must be held in strict confidence and that any use, release, or publication resulting therefrom must preclude identification of any person or persons studied. Violation of these statutes is a misdemeanor, and the violator may be civilly liable (*Id.* § 26-25-5).

Small healthcare facilities shall protect records against unauthorized access (*Id.* at 432-200-6.102) and keep records confidential (*Id.* at 432-200-6.103). Rules 432-201-4.201 and 432-201-4.203 establish similar rules for mental retardation facilities, as do rules 432-500-6.104 and 432-500-6.105 for freestanding ambulatory surgical centers and rules 432-600-6.104 and 432-600-6.105 for abortion clinics. Rules 432-550-8 and 432-650-3.206 provide that birthing centers and end-stage renal disease facilities, respectively, shall guard medical records against unauthorized access.

Home health agencies must develop policies that address confidentiality of medical records (*Id.* at 432-700-3.701 and 432-700-3.704). In addition, Rule 432-700-3.602 gives home health agency patients the right to be assured confidential treatment of personal and medical records, and to approve or refuse their release to any individual outside the agency, except in the case of transfer to another agency or health facility, or as provided by law or third-party payment contract.

Medical records and audits of HMOs are confidential (Utah Code Annotated § 31A-8-405), as is information involved in audits of HMOs (*Id.* § 31A-8-404).

Under the Medical Benefits Recovery Act, medical billing information is confidential (*Id.* § 26-19-18). Finally, § 31A-22-617 provides for confidentiality of information in medical records of patients during audits of preferred provider organizations.

Vermont

Vermont's Bill of Rights for Hospital Patients is contained in Vermont Statutes Annotated Title 18, § 1852, which states that patients have the right to expect that all communications and records pertaining to their care shall be treated as confidential. Only medical personnel or individuals under the supervision of medical personnel directly treating the patient, those persons monitoring the quality of that treatment, or researching the effectiveness of that treatment shall have access to the patient's medical records. Others may have access to those records only with the patient's written authorization. Vermont's physician-patient privilege amplifies the patient's rights to confidentiality by precluding disclosure of confidential information acquired by a healthcare practitioner in a professional capacity (*Id.* Title 12, § 1612).

Similarly, § 7301, the Nursing Home Residents' Bill of Rights, requires the staff of any facility to ensure that each person admitted to the facility is assured of confidential treatment of his or her personal and medical records, and the opportunity to approve or refuse their release to any individual outside the facility, except in case of his or her transfer to another healthcare institution or as required by law or third-party payment contract (*Id.* Title 33, § 7301).

Virginia

Department of Health, Rules and Regulations for the Licensure of Hospitals in Virginia Part III, § 208.6, specifies that medical records shall be kept confidential; that only authorized personnel shall have access to the records; and that the hospital shall release copies thereof only with the written consent of the patient, his or her legal representative, or to duly authorized state or federal health authorities or others authorized by the Virginia Code or federal statutes. If the patient is a minor, his or her parent, guardian, or legal representative must provide the consent. Under § 208.6.3, the hospital's permanent record may be removed from the hospital's jurisdiction only in accordance with a court order, subpoena, or statute. The same rules apply to nursing homes (Department of Health, Rules and Regulations for the Licensure of Nursing Homes in Virginia Part III, §§ 24.3 and 24.3.3).

Under § 32.1-138, patients in nursing homes are assured of confidential treatment of personal and medical records and may approve or refuse their release to any individual outside the facility, except in case of the patients' transfer to another healthcare institution or as required by law or third-party payment contract.

Washington

Revised Codes of Washington § 70.127.140 provides for patients' rights to have patient records treated confidentially by home health, hospice, and home care agencies.

Hospitals must establish policies and procedures that govern access to and release of data in patients' individual medical records and other medical data taking into consideration the confidential nature of these records (Washington Administrative Code § 248-18-440). These records and other personal or medical data on patients must be handled and stored so they are not accessible to unauthorized persons.

West Virginia

West Virginia Legislature, Title 64 West Virginia Legislative Rule 16-5C Department of the Board of Health, series 13, § 9.7, covers nursing home patients' rights to confidentiality. The rule states that patients are assured confidential treatment of their personal and healthcare records and condition. Such information shall not be discussed, without the patient's consent, with persons not treating or caring for the patient. A patient has the right to refuse release of his or her personal or healthcare records to any individual outside the facility, except as required by law or third-party payment contracts. A specific signed release by the patient is required for all other releases. A prior executed, blanket release is not acceptable.

Section 33-25A-26 makes confidential any data or information pertaining to the diagnosis, treatment, or health of any enrollee or applicant, that an HMO obtains from the person or a healthcare provider. Such information may not be disclosed except:

- As necessary to facilitate an assessment of the quality of care or to review the complaint system.
- Upon the express written consent of the enrollee or legally authorized representative.
- Pursuant to statute or court order.
- In the event of a claim or litigation between such person and the HMO in which such data or information is pertinent.

Further, the HMO may claim any privileges against disclosure which the provider could claim. (*Id.*).

Wisconsin

Under Wisconsin law, all healthcare records are confidential and may only be released upon informed consent or to those listed in Wisconsin Statutes § 146.82.

Wyoming

Wyoming Statutes § 35-2-609 provides that hospitals may not disclose any healthcare information about a patient to any other person without the patient's written authorization, except as authorized under § 35-2-606 (relating to disclosure to other providers who are providing care, for research, and so forth). Section 35-2-606(c) providing for such disclosure requires the receiver to use reasonable care to protect the confidentiality of the information.

Conclusion

Principles of medical ethics, physician-patient and similar privileges, and federal and state laws protect the confidentiality of medical information. Chapter 4 offers a discussion of enhanced confidentiality protection for certain categories of healthcare information.

4

Enhanced Confidentiality Protections

Introduction

As discussed in Chapter 3, patients have the right to confidentiality of medical records/information contained in medical ethics, in physician- and other professionals-patient privileges, and in government statutes and regulations. However, the law provides for additional protection for certain especially sensitive medical information, typically sexually transmitted or other communicable disease information, particularly HIV/AIDS information; alcohol and drug abuse information; and mental health/developmental disabilities information.

A patient's desire not to have a provider disclose that he or she has been diagnosed as HIV-positive or has received treatment for mental illness is understandable. Statutes providing for extra confidentiality protection for such sensitive information are based on the premise that the patient will not come forward for, say, HIV-testing unless the provider assures the patient of the confidentiality of the results. Cases are legion wherein patients lost their jobs, lost benefits, or suffered social stigma because of the improper disclosure of such sensitive information.

For example, in 1993, a New York appeals court ruled that a patient could recover punitive damages from a physician who disclosed that the patient was HIV-positive. The court noted that "the availability of punitive damages advances the New York Legislature's strong public policy protecting the confidentiality of a patient's HIV status and its condemnation of a breach of a physician's duty to protect confidentiality." [1]

The Joint Commission on Accreditation of Healthcare Organizations recognizes the need to provide for extra protection for such sensitive information in its Standard IM.2.2.2, which states that "[t]he organization has a functioning mechanism designed to preserve the confidentiality of data/information identified as sensitive or requiring extraordinary means to preserve patient privacy."[2] Thus, providers must be aware of and observe federal and state laws that provide for enhanced protection for sexually transmitted/communicable disease information, alcohol and drug abuse information, and mental health/developmental disabilities information.

Federal Laws

Federal statutes establish standards for disclosure of medical records of drug abusers. Violating patients' confidentiality may result in a criminal penalty. Under federal law, written consent must include the date, the names of the patient and the facility, the name of the party to whom the information may be disclosed, the purpose of the disclosure, the precise nature of the information to be disclosed, and the length of time the authorization is valid [42 United States Code § 242(a) (the Comprehensive Alcohol Abuse and Alcoholism Prevention, Treatment, and Rehabilitation Act of 1970); 42 United States Code § 290ee-2; 21 United States Code § 872(e) (as amended); 42 United States Code § 290ee-3 (transferred from 21 United States Code § 1175(b)(2)(c); a similar provision affects the Veterans Administration, 38 United States Code § 7333].

Any program relating to alcohol or drug abuse education, treatment, rehabilitation, or research that directly or indirectly receives federal assistance and that maintains records of the identity, diagnosis, or prognosis of any patient in connection with such programs must keep such records confidential (42 United States Code § 290dd-3).

Information on participants in an alcohol or drug program can be disclosed if the patient consents in writing, if there is an emergency situation in which medical history is necessary, for scientific research or other studies in which the individual will not be identified, or by court order.

Federal regulations require public, nonprofit, and for-profit private entities conducting, regulating, or assisting alcohol or drug abuse programs to maintain records showing patient consent to disclosure and documenting any disclosure, to medical personnel in a medical emergency, from confidential records (42 Code of Federal Regulations § 2.31-2.35 and 2.51-2.53). The regulation does not specify a retention period.

The federal regulations also require alcohol, drug abuse, and mental health researchers to maintain Confidentiality Certificates showing that the secretary of Health and Human Services has authorized the researcher to withhold the identity of research subjects in legal proceedings to compel the disclosure of the identity of research subjects, again without specifying a retention period (*Id.* § 2a-3 through 2a-8).

The provisions concerning confidentiality of drug and alcohol abuse patients are applicable to peer review organizations (*Id.* § 476.109).

Utilization review (UR) plans must provide that identities of individual recipients in all UR records and reports are kept confidential (*Id.* §§ 456.113, 456.213, and 456.313).

Section 417.115 outlines confidentiality requirements affecting federally qualified health maintenance organizations (HMOs). Each recipient of federal financial assistance must hold confidential all information obtained by its personnel about the participants in the project and must not disclose information, unless disclosure is authorized by the patient, necessary to treat the individual, required by law, or under compelling circumstances to protect the health or safety of an individual. However, information may be disclosed in summary, statistical, or other forms that do not identify individuals.

The Social Security Administration (SSA) and Health and Human Services Departments (HHS) release information held by them for research and statistical studies. The Privacy Act, 5 U.S.C. § 522a, allows disclosure of records held by these departments, but the records may not contain personal identifiers unless the identifiers are necessary for the research project and the department receives assurance from the requesting party of the privacy of the individuals under study. The departments will also release personal identifiers if the recipient guarantees the records' safety and submits to on-site inspection of those safeguards (20 C.F.R. § 401.325).

HHS also has procedures to protect the privacy of research subjects in federally funded research studies [*Id.* (found at 45 C.F.R. § 46.102 *et seq.*)].

State Laws

States usually provide for enhanced protection for sexually transmitted/communicable disease information, alcohol and drug abuse information, and mental health information.

Alabama

Reports of sexually transmitted disease are confidential, and anyone who makes an unauthorized release is guilty of a misdemeanor *(Id.* § 22-11A-14).

Alabama has no specific requirements for alcohol and drug abuse records over and above the federal requirements.

Under Alabama Code § 22-50-62, no employee of any of the facilities under the management, control, supervision, or affiliation of the Alabama Department of Mental Health and Mental Retardation shall be required to disclose any record, report, case history, memorandum, or other information, oral or written, that may have been acquired, made, or compiled in attending or treating any patient of said facilities in a professional character, when such information was necessary in order to evaluate or treat said patient or to do any act for him or her in a professional capacity, except when:

- A court of competent jurisdiction shall order disclosure for the promotion of justice.
- The court orders a mental examination of a defendant in a criminal case.

Alaska

Under Alaska Statutes § 47.37.210, the registration and other records of alcohol and intoxication treatment facilities are confidential and are privileged to the patient, except they may be used for purposes of research into the causes and treatment of alcoholism. No information may disclose a patient's name.

Under Alaska Statutes § 47.30.590, mental health records are confidential and must be safeguarded.

Arizona

Communicable disease information is confidential (Arizona Revised Statute § 36-664). Arizona provides detailed guidance concerning to whom a practitioner may release such information, including:

- The protected person or, if the protected person lacks capacity to consent, a person authorized by law to consent.
- Agents or employees of health facilities or providers, if the agents or employees are authorized to access medical records, if the facilities or providers are authorized to obtain such information, and if the agents or employees provide healthcare to the protected individual or maintain or possess medical records for billing or reimbursement.
- Healthcare providers or facilities, if knowledge of the communicable disease-related information is necessary to provide appropriate care or treatment to the person or a child.
- Health facilities or providers in relation to the procurement, processing, distributing, or use of a human body or a human body part, including fluids, for use in medical education, research, or therapy, or for transport to another person.
- A peer review, utilization review, or similar activity, so long as the disclosure does not include information directly identifying the protected person.
- Federal, state, county, or local health officers, if disclosure is mandated by law.
- Government agencies authorized by law to receive the information.

Information may also be released pursuant to a court order or a written release, if any of the following conditions exist:

- Disclosure is authorized by law.
- Disclosure is made to a contact of the protected person.
- Disclosure is made pursuant to a release of confidential communicable disease information.
- Disclosure is for the purpose of research (*Id.*).

Any disclosure made pursuant to a release must be accompanied by a statement in writing that warns that the information is from confidential records and protected by state law that prohibits further disclosure without the specific written consent of the person to whom it pertains or as otherwise permitted by law. The person making a disclosure must keep a record of all disclosures.

Under Arizona Revised Statutes, tuberculosis control officers may, with the consent of the attending physician, examine any and all records, reports, and other data pertaining to the tuberculosis condition of tuberculosis patients, but information so obtained is confidential, privileged, and cannot be divulged so as to disclose the identity of the person to whom it relates (*Id.* § 36-714).

Arizona Revised Statutes § 32-1457 provides a limited exception to the confidentiality of HIV/AIDS information by permitting disclosure to others endangered by the patient under certain circumstances.

Arizona statutes regarding mental health services state that all information and records obtained in the course of evaluation, examination, or treatment must be kept confidential and not as public records, except when the requirements of a hearing pursuant to these statutes necessitate a different procedure [Arizona Revised Statutes § 36-509 (A)]. Information and records may only be disclosed pursuant to rules established by the department to:

- Physicians and providers of health, mental health, social, and welfare services involved in caring, treating, or rehabilitating the patient.

- Individuals to whom the patient has given consent to have information disclosed.

- Persons legally representing the patient (in such cases, the department's rules may not delay complete disclosure).

- Persons authorized by a court order.

- Persons doing research or maintaining health statistics, provided the department establishes rules for the conduct of such research to ensure the anonymity of the patient.

- State department of corrections in cases where prisoners confined to the state prison are patients in the state hospital on authorized transfer either by voluntary admission or by order of the court.

- Governmental or law enforcement agencies when necessary to secure the return of a patient who is on unauthorized absence from any agency where the patient was undergoing evaluation and treatment.

- Family members actively participating in the patient's care, treatment, or supervision. An agency or treating professional may only release information relating to the person's diagnosis, prognosis, need for hospitalization, anticipated length of stay, discharge plan, medication, medication side effects, and short-term and long-term treatment goals (*Id.*).

An agency may release information under this statute only after the treating professional or professional's designee interviews the person undergoing treatment or evaluation to determine whether release is in that person's best interests. A decision to release or withhold information is subject to review pursuant to the law [*Id.* § 36-509(B) (pursuant to § 36-517.01)]. The treating agency must record the name of any person to whom information is given.

The definition of unprofessional practice for psychotherapists includes betraying a professional confidence (*Id.* § 32-3251).

Arkansas

All laboratory notifications of communicable diseases are confidential and shall not be open to inspection by anyone except public health personnel (Arkansas Code Annotated § 20-16-504).

In addition, *Id.* § 20-15-901 provides that the identification of persons voluntarily participating in the Department of Health AIDS testing program must be kept secret.

A patient has a privilege to refuse to disclose and to prevent any other from disclosing confidential communications made for the purpose of diagnosis or treatment of his or her physical, mental, or emotional condition, including alcohol or drug addiction (*Id.* § 16-41-101).

California

California Health and Safety Code § 199.21 provides for both civil and criminal liability for wrongful disclosure of AIDS test results. Any person who negligently discloses results of an HIV test to any third party, in a manner that identifies or provides identifying characteristics of the person to whom the test results apply, except pursuant to a written authorization or as otherwise authorized by law, shall be assessed a civil penalty in an amount not to exceed $1,000 plus court costs. Any person who willfully discloses the results of an HIV test to any third party, in a manner that identifies or provides identifying characteristics of the person to whom the test results apply, except pursuant to a written authorization or as authorized by law, shall be assessed a civil penalty in an amount not less than $1,000 and not more than $5,000 plus court costs.

Any person who willfully or negligently discloses the results of an HIV test to a third party, in a manner that identifies or provides identifying characteristics of the person to whom the test results apply—except pursuant to a written authorization, or as authorized by law—which results in economic, bodily, or psychological harm to the subject of the test is guilty of a misdemeanor, punishable by imprisonment in the county jail for a period not to exceed one year or a fine of not to exceed $10,000 or both.

Any person who commits any act just described shall be liable to the subject for all actual damages, including damages for economic, bodily, or psychological harm that is a proximate result of the act. Each disclosure made in violation of this chapter is a separate and actionable offense.

"Written authorization" applies only to the disclosure of test results by a person responsible for the care and treatment of the person subject to the test. Written authorization is required for each separate disclosure of the test results and shall include to whom the disclosure would be made.

However, nothing in this statute imposes liability or criminal sanction for disclosure of an HIV test in accordance with any reporting requirement for a diagnosed case of AIDS by the State Department or the Centers for Disease Control under the United States Public Health Service.

The State Department may require blood banks and plasma centers to submit monthly reports summarizing statistical data concerning the results of tests to detect the presence of viral hepatitis and HIV. This statistical summary shall not include the identity of individual donors or identifying characteristics that would identify individual donors.

Disclosed, as used in this statute, means to disclose, release, transfer, disseminate, or otherwise communicate all or any part of any record orally, in writing, or by electronic means to any person or entity.

When the results of an HIV test are included in the medical record of the patient who is the subject of the test, the inclusion is not a disclosure for purposes of this section.

Notwithstanding § 199.21, the results of an HIV test that identifies or provides identifying characteristics of the person to whom the test results apply may be recorded by the physician who ordered the test in the test subject's medical record or otherwise disclosed without written authorization of the subject of the test, or the subject's representative, to the test subject's providers of health care, for purpose of diagnosis, care, or treatment of the patient, except that for purposes of this section *providers of health care* do not include a health care service plan. Recording or disclosure of HIV test results pursuant to this statute does not authorize further disclosure unless otherwise permitted by law (*Id.* § 199.215).

Section 199.30 provides for confidentiality of research records of AIDS patients. *Id.* § 199.32 states that such records must be protected in the course of conducting financial audits or program evaluations, and audit personnel shall not directly or indirectly identify any individual research subject in any report of a financial audit or program evaluation. To the extent it is necessary for audit personnel to know the identity of individual research subjects, authorized disclosure of confidential research records shall be made on a case-by-case basis, and every prudent effort shall be exercised to safeguard the confidentiality of these research records in accordance with this chapter. Information disclosed for audit or evaluation purposes should be used only for audit and evaluation purposes and may not be redisclosed or used in any other way.

Individuals or entities treating or rehabilitating patients impaired by drug or alcohol abuse must keep records of such treatment confidential (California Business and Professions Code § 156.1). California Health and Safety Code adds that the identity and records of the identity, diagnosis, prognosis, or treatment of any narcotics or drug abuse treatment or prevention patient are confidential and may only be disclosed under the limited circumstances authorized by the statute. In addition, California Civil Code § 56.30 specifies that California providers must follow the federal alcohol and drug abuse regulations.

Similarly, the Welfare and Institutions Code § 5328 covers psychiatric records. In such cases, patient authorization requires the approval of a physician, psychologist, or social worker. Mandatory disclosure is required:

- Between qualified professionals when providing services, in referrals, and in conservatorship hearings.
- To the extent necessary to make an insurance claim.
- To persons designated by the conservator.
- For research.
- To courts and law enforcement agencies as needed to protect public officials.
- To the patient's attorney.
- To probation officers.
- To patients' rights advocates with patient authorization.
- To law enforcement officials if the patient is a victim or has committed a crime in the facility.

Whenever a facility discloses such information, the facility shall promptly cause to be entered into the patient's medical record: the date and circumstances under which such disclosure was made; the names and relationships to the patient if any, of persons or agencies to whom such disclosure was made; and the specific information disclosed (*Id.* § 5328.06).

Permissive disclosure of information, not access to the records, is allowed to the family or persons designated by the patient or without designation if the patient is unable to give consent.

Section 4514 has similar provisions for records of the developmentally disabled. Facilities must record the circumstances of the disclosure in the patient's record (*Id.* § 4516).

Colorado

Colorado does not permit a person responsible for the diagnosis or treatment of venereal diseases of a minor or his or her addiction to or use of drugs to release records of such diagnosis or treatment to the parent, guardian, or other person other than the minor or his or her designated representative [Colorado Revised Statutes § 25-1-801(d)].

The registration and other records of drug abusers are confidential. Colorado requires treatment facilities to protect such records as required by the federal confidentiality regulations (Colorado Revised Statutes § 25-1-1108).

Section 27-10-120 provides that records pertaining to the care and treatment of the mentally ill are confidential.

Connecticut

Under Connecticut General Statute § 19a-583, no person may disclose HIV-related information except to the following:

- The protected individual or legal guardian.

- Any person who secures a release of confidential HIV-related information.

- Federal, state, or local health officers, when such disclosure is mandated or authorized by federal or state law.

- Healthcare provider or health facilities when knowledge of the HIV-related information is necessary to provide appropriate care or treatment to the protected individual or a child or when confidential HIV-related information is already recorded in a medical chart or record and a healthcare provider has access to such record for the purpose of providing medical care to the protected individual.

- Medical examiner to assist in determining the cause or circumstances of death.

- Health facility staff committees or accreditation or oversight review organizations that are conducting program monitoring, program evaluation, or service reviews.

- Healthcare provider or other person in cases where such person in the course of his or her occupational duties has had significant exposure to HIV infection, providing detailed criteria are met.
- Employees of hospitals for mental illness operated by the Department of Mental Health, if the infection control committee of the hospital determines that the behavior of the patient poses a significant risk of transmission to another patient and specific criteria are met.
- Employees of facilities operated by the Department of Correction, if specific criteria are met.
- By court order, which is issued in compliance with the following provisions:
  - The court finds a clear and imminent danger to the public health or the health of a person and that the person has demonstrated a compelling need for the test results that cannot be accommodated by other means.
  - Pleadings pertaining to disclosure of confidential HIV-related information substitute a pseudonym for the true name of the subject of the test.
  - Before granting any such order, the court provides the individual whose test result is in question with notice and a reasonable opportunity to participate in the proceedings.
  - The court proceedings are conducted *in camera* unless the subject of the test agrees to a hearing in open court or unless the court determines that a public hearing is necessary to the public interest and the proper administration of justice.
  - Upon the issuance of an order to disclose test results, the court imposes appropriate safeguards against unauthorized disclosure, which must specify the persons who may have access to the information, the purposes for which the information must be used, and appropriate prohibitions on future disclosure.
- Life and health insurers, government payers, and healthcare centers and their affiliates, reinsurers, and contractors (except agents and brokers) in connection with underwriting and claim activity for life, health, and disability benefits.
- Any healthcare provider specifically designated by the protected individual to receive such information received by a life or health

insurer or healthcare center pursuant to an application for life, health, or disability insurance (*Id.*).

Whenever confidential HIV-related information is disclosed, it must be accompanied by a statement in writing, whenever possible, that includes the following or substantially similar language:

This information has been disclosed to you from records whose confidentiality is protected by state law. State law prohibits you from making any further disclosure of it without the specific written consent of the person to whom it pertains, or as otherwise permitted by said law. A general authorization for the release of medical or other information is *not* sufficient for this purpose (*Id.* § 19a-585).

A notation of all permitted disclosures should be placed in the medical record.

Information showing that a doctor consulted with, examined, or treated a minor for venereal disease is confidential (*Id.* § 19a-216.)

Section 17a-630 provides for maintaining the confidentiality of alcohol and drug abuse patients. Records of applicants for enrollment and enrolled patients in community drug abuse treatment programs are confidential [*Id.* § 17a-630(b)-(c)], as are records showing that a minor requested or received treatment and rehabilitation for drug dependence [*Id.* § 17a-630(d)].

The commissioner of mental health is responsible for ensuring maximum safeguards of mental health patient confidentiality (Connecticut General Statutes § 17a-451). Section 52-146d makes communications between psychiatrists and patients privileged.

Delaware

Information and records held by the Division of Public Health relating to known or suspected sexually transmitted diseases, including HIV infection, are confidential, as are reports of venereal disease cases (*Id.* § 702), and may only be released in limited circumstances (*Id.* Title 16, §§ 711 & 712).

Delaware Code Title 16, § 1203 authorizes disclosure of HIV tests to health facility staff committees or accreditation or oversight review organizations that are conducting program monitoring, program evaluation, or service reviews.

Information and records held by the Division of Public Health relating to known or suspected sexually transmitted diseases, including HIV infection, are confidential and may only be released if release is made:

- Of medical or epidemiological information for statistical purposes so that no person can be identified.

- Of medical or epidemiological information with the consent of all persons identified in the information released.

- Of medical or epidemiological information to medical personnel, appropriate state agencies, or state courts to the extent required to enforce the provisions of the law and related rules and regulations concerning the control and treatment of sexually transmitted diseases, or as related to child abuse investigation.

- Of medical or epidemiological information to medical personnel in a medical emergency to the extent necessary to protect the health or life of a named party.

- During the course of civil or criminal litigation to a person allowed access to said records by a court order issued in compliance with the detailed requirements of the law (Delaware Code Annotated Title 16, §§ 711-712 or 702).

Violations of these reporting requirements may result in a fine of between $100 and $1,000 [*Id.* § 713(a) (this section does not cover reporting of sexually transmitted diseases)]. A violation of this law and the law concerning reporting of sexually transmitted diseases may result in a fine of $25 to $200 (*Id.* §§ 713 and 702).

No person may disclose or be compelled to disclose the identity of any person upon whom an HIV-related test is performed or the results of such test in a manner that permits identification of the subject of the test, except to the following persons (*Id.* § 1203):

- The subject of the test or subject's legal guardian.

- Any person who secures a legally effective release of test results executed by the subject of the test or subject's legal guardian.

- An authorized agent or employee of a healthcare facility or healthcare provider, if the health facility or provider itself is authorized to obtain the test results, if the agent or employee provides patient care or handles or processes specimens of body fluids or tissues, and the agent or employee has a medical need to know such information to provide health care to the patient.

- Healthcare providers providing medical care to the subject of the test, when knowledge of test results is necessary to provide appropriate medical care or treatment.

- State review staff when part of an official report to the Division of Public Health, as may be required by regulation.

- A health facility or healthcare provider that procures, processes, distributes or uses:

  - Blood.

  - Human body part from a deceased person donated for a purpose specified under the Uniform Anatomical Gift Act.

  - Semen provided prior to July 11, 1988, for the purpose of artificial insemination.

  - Health facility staff committees or accreditation or oversight review organizations that are conducting program monitoring, program evaluation, or service reviews.

- Those investigating suspected instances of child abuse (*Id.* §§ 901-909.

- People seeking to control sexually transmitted diseases (*Id.* §§ 701-713).

- Those handling a court order issued in compliance with the detailed requirements of the statute (*Id.* § 1203).

Anyone aggrieved by an improper disclosure of such information may recover damages of $1,000 or actual damages, whichever is greater, if the violation is negligent; damages of $5,000 or actual damages, if the violation is intentional or reckless; and reasonable attorney's fees and other relief, such as an injunction, that the court deems appropriate [*Id.* § 1204(a)].

The registration and other records of alcoholism and intoxication treatment facilities shall remain confidential in accordance with the federal requirements at 42 C.F.R., Part II, and are privileged to the patient (16 Delaware Code § 2214).

Clinical records of mental health patients (*Id.* Title 16, § 5161) and health information obtained by HMOs (*Id.* Title 16, § 9113) are confidential.

District of Columbia

Records related to a case of communicable, environmentally or occupationally related disease or medical condition may be used for statistical and public health purposes only. Any identifying information in the records may be disclosed only when necessary to safeguard the physical health of others. No person is allowed to disclose or redisclose identifying information from such records unless the patient gives prior written permission or a court finds, on clear and convincing evidence, that the disclosure is necessary to safeguard another's health or to provide evidence probative of guilt or innocence in a criminal prosecution (District of Columbia Code Annotated § 6-117).

The administrator of Preventive Health Services Administration, Commission on Public Health, Department of Human Services, is authorized to make any necessary investigation to determine the source of the infection and the nature of treatment. Hospitals, laboratories, and physicians are required to make medical records and histories available to the administrator to facilitate such investigations. The administrator, however, may not disclose the identity of an AIDS patient without that person's written permission.

The provisions of the Preventive Health Services Amendments Act of 1985 pertaining to the confidentiality of medical records and information on persons with AIDS, apply to AIDS treatment (*Id.* § 6-2805).

Other than the general federal rules, D.C. statutes provide that the registration and other records of a detoxification center shall remain confidential and may be disclosed only to medical personnel for purposes of diagnosis, treatment, and court testimony; to police personnel for purposes of investigation of criminal offenses and complaints against police action; and to authorized personnel for purposes of presentence reports (*Id.* § 24-524).

Section 6-2002 prohibits disclosure of mental health information by any mental health professional or facility to any person, including an employer.

Florida

Under Florida Statutes § 381.004, HIV test results are confidential. No person who has obtained or has knowledge of a test result pursuant to this section may disclose or be compelled to disclose the identity of any person upon whom a test is performed, or the results of such a test in a manner that permits identification of the subject of the test, with limited exceptions.

Florida Statutes chapter 381.004(8) allows disclosure of HIV test results to authorized medical or epidemiological researchers, who may not further disclose any identifying characteristics or information.

Florida Statutes § 112.0455 makes confidential all information, interviews, reports, statements, memoranda, and drug test results, written or otherwise, of drug testing programs. Employers, laboratories, employee assistance programs, drug and alcohol rehabilitation programs, and their agents who receive or have access to information concerning drug test results shall keep all information confidential and may release it only upon consent or in other limited circumstances.

The rights of mental health patients include confidentiality of clinical records. Unless waived by express and informed consent, the confidential status of such clinical records shall not be lost by either authorized or unauthorized disclosure to any person, organization, or agency. The facility may not release any part of the clinical record except in the limited circumstances authorized by the statute (Florida Statutes § 394.459). Section 455.2415 adds that communications between patients and psychiatrists are confidential and may not be disclosed except at the request of the patient or the patient's legal representative.

Insurers must maintain strict confidentiality regarding psychiatric and psychotherapeutic records submitted for the purpose of reviewing a claim for benefits (Florida Statutes § 627.668).

The investigations, proceedings, and records of a peer review committee are not subject to discovery or introduction into evidence in any civil or administrative action against a provider of professional health services arising out of the matters that are the subject of evaluation and review by such committee. However, information, documents, or records otherwise available from original sources are not to be construed as immune from discovery or use in any such civil action merely because they were presented during proceedings of such committee (Florida Statutes § 766.101).

Georgia

Georgia Code section 24-9-47 makes AIDS information confidential and specifies the limited circumstances under which such information may be disclosed.

Section 26-5-17 provides for confidentiality of records, names, and communications of drug-dependent persons who seek or obtain treatment, therapeutic advice, or counsel from any licensed program. Further, any communication such person has with an authorized employee or license holder is confidential.

Mental health records are covered by Georgia's general mental record confidentiality statute, § 37-3-166, and by physician- or psychologist-patient privileges, §§ 24-9-21(5) and 43-39-16. *See Annandale at Suwanee, Inc. v. Weatherly,* 194 Ga. App. 803, 392 S.E.2d 27 (1990).

Hawaii

Hawaii provides for confidentiality in reports of communicable diseases by prohibiting disclosures that would identify the persons to whom the records relate, except as necessary to safeguard the public health against those who disobey the rules relating to such diseases (*Id.* § 325-4). The confidentiality of HIV infection, ARC, and AIDS records information is assured, and related information may not be released or made public upon subpoena or any other method of discovery [*Id.* § 325-101(a)]. However, release of this information is permitted if:

- Release is made to the Department of Health in order to comply with federal reporting requirements imposed on the state. The department must ensure that personal identifying information from these records is protected from public disclosure.

- Release is made of the records, or of specific medical or epidemiological information contained therein, with the prior written consent of the person or persons to whom the records pertain.

- Release is made to medical personnel in a medical emergency only to the extent necessary to protect the health, life, or well-being of the named party.

- Release to or by the Department of Health is necessary to protect the health and well-being of the general public, provided such release is made in such a way that no person can be identified, except as specified in law.

- Release is made by the Department of Health of medical or epidemiological information from the records to medical personnel, appropriate county and state agencies, blood banks, plasma centers, organ and tissue banks, schools, preschools, day care centers, or county or district courts to enforce this part and to enforce rules adopted by the Department of Health concerning the control and treatment of HIV infection, ARC, and AIDS, provided that release of information is only made by confidential communication to a designated individual.

- Release of a child's records is made to the Department of Human Services for the purpose of enforcing child abuse laws or suspect transmission of the HIV virus.

- Release of a child's records is made within the Department of Human Services and to child protective services team consultants under contract to the Department of Human Services for the purpose of enforcing and administering the law on a need-to-know basis pursuant to a written protocol to be established and implemented, in consultation with the director of health, by the director of human services.

- Release of a child's records is made by employees of the Department of Human Services authorized to do so by the protocol established in the law to a natural parent of a child who is the subject of the case when the natural parent is a client in the case, the guardian *ad litem* of the child, the court, each party to the court proceedings, and also to an adoptive or a prospective adoptive parent, an individual or an agency with whom the child is placed for 24-hour residential care, and medical personnel responsible for the care or treatment of the child. When a release is made to a natural parent of the child, it must be with appropriate counseling as required by the law [*Id.* § 325-101(b) (see section 325-16)]. In no event may proceedings be initiated against a child's natural parents for claims of child abuse or harm to a child or to affect parental rights solely on the basis of the HIV seropositivity of a child or of the child's natural parents.

- Release is made to the patient's healthcare insurer to obtain reimbursement for services rendered to the patient; provided that release will not be made if, after being informed that a claim will be made to an insurer, the patient is afforded the opportunity to make the reimbursement directly and actually makes the reimbursement.

- Release is made by the patient's healthcare provider to another healthcare provider for the purpose of continued care or treatment of the patient.

- Release is made pursuant to a court order, after an *in camera* review of the records, upon a showing of good cause by the party seeking the release of the records (*Id.*).

Hawaii's evidence code makes communications for the purpose of diagnosis and treatment of physical, mental, or emotional conditions, including alcohol or drug addiction, privileged and confidential (Hawaii Revised Statutes § 504).

Hawaii's evidence code makes communications for the purpose of diagnosis and treatment of mental conditions and between psychiatrists and patients privileged and confidential (*Id.*).

Idaho

All reports of reportable diseases made to the Department of Health and Welfare are confidential (Idaho Code § 39-606). Confidential disease reports containing patient identification reported under the statute may be only used by public health officials who must conduct investigations and may be disclosed only as provided by law. Any person who willfully or maliciously discloses the content of any of these confidential public health records is guilty of a misdemeanor (*Id.*).

Section 39-308 makes records of treatment facilities for alcoholism confidential and privileged to the patient.

The Idaho statute providing for immunity from liability for warning third parties of a mental health patient's violent behavior states that no professional disciplinary procedure, monetary liability, or cause of action may arise for disclosing confidential or privileged information in an effort to so warn others (Idaho Code § 6-1904).

Illinois

Illinois requires strict confidentiality for reporting of communicable diseases, including sexually transmissible diseases 745 (ILCS 45/1).

Reports of incidents of sexually transmitted diseases, including AIDS, to the Public Health Department are confidential, but may be disclosed:

- With consent.

- For statistical purposes and medical or epidemiologic information, if summarized so no one can be identified and no names are revealed.

- When made to medical personnel, appropriate state agencies, or courts to enforce the statute.

- When pursuant to a subpoena, in such cases, the information must be sealed by the court, except as necessary to reach a decision or as otherwise agreed by all parties; and the proceedings must be *in camera* and the record sealed (410 Illinois Compiled Statutes 3251).

- When authorized by the AIDS Confidentiality Act [Illinois Administrative Code Title 77, § 693.100(b)(5); *see also* 410 Illinois Compiled Statutes 305/15].

- When made to a school principal [Illinois Administrative Code Title 77, § 693.100(b)(6)].

- When authorized by the AIDS Registry System Regulations [Illinois Administrative Code Title 77, § 693.100(b)(4)].

Insurance companies and health services corporations that require patients or applicants for new or continued coverage to be tested for AIDS must keep the results confidential (410 Illinois Compiled Statutes 50/3).

Illinois law requires keeping drug and alcohol abuse patient records strictly confidential (20 ILCS 305/8-102).

The Mental Health and Developmental Disabilities Confidentiality Act prohibits disclosure that a named person is a recipient of mental health care (735 ILCS 110/2 *et seq.*).

Indiana

Indiana Code §§ 16-4-9-5 through 16-4-9-8 provide for the confidentiality of information for cancer research purposes. Generally, any disclosure cannot identify individual patients.

Communicable or other disease information is confidential, but disclosure is permitted for statistical purposes if done in a manner that does not identify any individual, with the individual's consent, or to the extent necessary to enforce public health laws or to protect the life or health of a third party.

Section 16-1-9.5-2 prohibits the inclusion of the name or other identifying characteristics of the individual tested for HIV or AIDS in a report. The board may adopt rules under § 4-22-2 concerning the compilation for statistical purposes of other information collected under this section.

Section 16-41-2-3 permits reporting HIV infection that does not involve a confirmed case of AIDS, to the State Medical Board if:

- The individual is enrolled in a formal research project for which a written study protocol has been filed with the state board.

- An individual is tested anonymously at a designated counseling or testing site.

- An individual who is tested by a healthcare provider is permitted by rule by the State Medical Board to use a number identifier code.

Such report may not include the name or other identifying characteristics of the person tested.

Section 16-1-9.5-7(a) provides that a person may not disclose or be compelled to disclose medical or epidemiological information involving a communicable disease or other disease that is a danger to general health. This information may not be released or made public upon subpoena or otherwise, except under the following circumstances:

- Release may be made of medical or epidemiologic information for statistical purposes if done in a manner that does not identify any individual.

- Release may be made of medical or epidemiologic information with the written consent of all individuals identified in the information released.

- Release may be made of medical or epidemiologic information to the extent necessary to enforce public health laws, to comply with laws described in section 35-38-1-7,[3] or to protect the health or life of a named party.

Further, release of such information is prohibited unless:

- Release shall be made of the medical records concerning an individual to that individual or to a person authorized in writing by that individual to receive the medical records *[Id.* § 16-1-9-7(d)].
- An individual may voluntarily disclose information about that individual's communicable disease (*Id.* § 16-1-9.5-9).

Any person responsible for recording, reporting, or maintaining information required to be reported under this section who recklessly, knowingly, or intentionally discloses or fails to protect medical or epidemiological information classified as confidential under this section commits a Class A misdemeanor. In addition, any public employee who violates this section is subject to discharge or other disciplinary action under the personnel rules of that governmental agency [*Id.* § 16-9.5-7(c) and (e)].

Indiana follows the federal rules on alcohol and drug abuse patient records. (*See* Indiana Code § 16-4-8-3.2.)

Indiana Code §§ 16-4-8-3.1 and 3.2 contain detailed rules for the disclosure of mental health records. Except for authorized disclosures, such records are not discoverable or admissible in any legal proceeding without the patient's consent. Section 25-33-1-17 specifies that communications between psychologists and clients are privileged.

Iowa

Reports on AIDS are confidential, and information in such reports may not be released except under the following circumstances (Iowa Code § 141.10):

- Medical or epidemiological information may be released for statistical purposes, in a manner such that no individual person can be identified.
- Medical or epidemiological information may be released to the extent necessary to enforce the provisions of the statute and related rules concerning the treatment, control, and investigation of the HIV infection by public health officials.
- Medical or epidemiological information may be released to medical personnel in a medical emergency to the extent necessary to protect the health or life of the named party.

- Test results concerning a patient may be released pursuant to procedures established under the Iowa code *(Id.)*.

Iowa permits disclosure of otherwise-confidential HIV information to protect a third party from the direct risk of transmission after making a reasonable attempt to warn, in writing, the infected person of the nature of and reason for the disclosure, the date of disclosure, and the name of the party or parties to whom the disclosure is to be made [*Id.* § 141.6(2)(d)(2)].

Communicable disease reports are also confidential (*Id.* § 139.2).

Section 125.93 makes involuntary commitment or treatment of substance abusers' records confidential, consistent with the federal confidentiality laws.

Section 229.25 requires hospitals or other facilities treating mentally ill persons to keep records relating to the examination, custody, care, and treatment of any person in that hospital or facility confidential, with three exceptions:

- When the information is requested by a licensed physician, attorney, or advocate who provides the facility's chief medical officer with a written waiver signed by the patient.

- When the information is sought by a court order.

- When the person who is hospitalized or the patient's guardian, if the person is a minor or is not legally competent, signs an informed consent release specifying the person or agency to whom the facility is to send the information.

The chief medical officer may release such records for research purposes so long as he or she does not disclose patients' names or identities. The officer may also release appropriate information to the spouse of a patient if the officer deems it to be in the best interests of the patient and the spouse.

Rule 481-63.38(135C) guarantees residents of residential care facilities for the mentally handicapped confidential treatment of all information contained in their medical, personal, and financial records.

The interpretive guidelines to the regulations governing confidentiality of mentally retarded patient records [*Id.* § 483.410(c)(1)] defines *keep confidential* as safeguarding the content of information including video, audio, and/or computer-stored information from unauthorized disclosure without the specific informed consent of the individual, parent of a minor child, or legal guardian, and consistent with the advocate's right of access as required in the Developmental Disabilities Act. If the facility maintains information that is too confidential to place in the record used by all staff, it may retain the information in a secure place and make a notation in the record of the location of confidential record.

Kansas

Information required to be reported and information obtained through laboratory tests conducted by the Department of Health and Environment relating to HIV or AIDS and persons suffering from or infected with HIV or AIDS is confidential and may not be disclosed beyond the disclosure necessary to comply with the law, Kansas Statute Annotated § 65-6003(a), or the usual reporting of laboratory test results to persons specifically designated by the secretary as authorized to obtain such information. Such information may be disclosed, however, under the following circumstances:

- No person can be identified in the information to be disclosed and the disclosure is for statistical purposes.

- All persons who are identifiable in the information to be disclosed consent in writing to its disclosure.

- Disclosure is necessary, and only to the extent necessary to protect public health, as specified by rules and regulations of the secretary.

- A medical emergency exists and disclosure is to medical personnel qualified to treat AIDS, but only to the extent necessary to protect the health or life of a named party.

- Information to be disclosed is required in a court proceeding involving a minor and the information is disclosed in camera [*Id.* §§ 65-6002(c) and 65-6003(b)].

The Secretary of Health and Environment may adopt and enforce rules and regulations for the prevention and control of AIDS and for such other measures as may be necessary to protect the public health [*Id.* § 65-6003(a)]. Physicians are authorized to disclose that a patient has AIDS or has had a positive reaction to an AIDS test to other healthcare providers who will be placed in contact with bodily fluids of such patient during such procedures. Such information is otherwise confidential [*Id.* § 65-6004(a)].

Public agencies are not required to disclose alcoholism or drug-dependency treatment records that pertain to identifiable patients (Kansas Statutes § 45-221).

An alcoholism or drug-dependency treatment facility may not disclose that a patient is or has been receiving treatment or any confidential communications made for the purposes of diagnosis or treatment (*Id.* § 65-5602).

Public agencies are not required to disclose psychiatric or psychological treatment records that pertain to identifiable patients (*Id.* § 45-221).

A mental health treatment facility may not disclose that a patient is or has been receiving treatment or any confidential communications made for the purposes of diagnosis or treatment (*Id.* § 65-5602).

Section 74-5323 provides for a psychologist-client privilege.

Section 74-5515 provides for confidentiality of records of developmental disability protection and advocacy agencies.

Kentucky

All records in the possession of local health departments or the Cabinet for Human Resources that concern persons infected with sexually transmitted diseases are confidential and may only be released to the physician retained by the patient, for statistical purposes as long as no individual can be identified, with consent, if necessary to enforce the rules of the cabinet for human resources relating to the control and treatment of such diseases, and to the extent necessary to protect the life or health of the named party [Kentucky Revised Statutes Annotated § 214.420(2)].

Administrators of alcoholism treatment and rehabilitation facilities must keep treatment records confidential (*Id.* § 222.270).

Information provided to the Cabinet for Human Resources relating to the effectiveness of chemical dependency treatment is confidential with respect to the identity of individual clients (*Id.* § 222.460).

Under Kentucky Revised Statutes § 202A.991, a person who violates the confidentiality of any mental health record is guilty of a misdemeanor.

All applications and requests for admission and release, and all certifications, records, and reports of the Cabinet for Human Resources that directly or indirectly identify a patient or former patient or a person whose hospitalization has been sought are confidential (*Id.* § 210.235).

Kentucky law provides for a psychotherapist-patient privilege (*Id.* § 422A.0507).

Louisiana

A patient requesting the performance of an HIV-related test shall be provided an opportunity to remain anonymous by the use of a coded system with no correlation or identification of the individual's identity to the specific test request or results. A healthcare provider that is not able to provide HIV-related tests on an anonymous basis shall refer, at no extra charge to the individual seeking anonymity, such individual to a test site that does provide anonymous testing. The provisions of this statute shall not apply to inpatients in hospitals (Louisiana Revised Statutes § 1300.13).

Except as otherwise provided by law, no person who obtains, retains, or becomes the recipient of confidential HIV test results in the course of providing any health or social service or pursuant to a release of confidential HIV test results may disclose such information pursuant to a written authorization to release medical information when such authorization contains a refusal to release HIV test results.

Notwithstanding the preceding, HIV test results may be released to the following:

- Any person to whom disclosure of medical information is authorized by law without the consent of the patient.
- Any agent or employee of a health facility or healthcare provider if :
  - The agent or employee is permitted access to medical records.
  - The health facility or healthcare provider is authorized to obtain the HIV test results.
  - The agent or employee provides health care to the patient or maintains or processes medical records for billing or reimbursement purposes.
- A healthcare provider or health facility, when knowledge of the HIV test results is necessary to provide appropriate care or treatment to the patient and afford the healthcare provider and the personnel of the health facility an opportunity to protect themselves from transmission of the virus.
- A health facility or healthcare provider, in relation to the procurement, processing, distributing, or use of a human body or a human body part, including organs, tissues, eyes, bones, arteries, blood, semen, or other body fluids, for use in medical education, research, therapy, or transplantation.
- Any health facility staff committees or accreditation or oversight review organizations authorized to access medical records, provided that the committee or organization shall only disclose confidential HIV test results:
  - To the facility or provider of a health or social service.
  - To a federal, state, or local government agency for the purposes of and subject to the conditions provided in the next item.

- To carry out the monitoring evaluation or service for which it was obtained.

- A federal, state, parish, or local health officer when the disclosure is mandated by federal or state law.

- An agency or individual in connection with the foster care programs of the Department of Social Services or an agency or individual in connection with the adoption of a child.

- Any person to whom disclosure is ordered by a court of competent jurisdiction.

- An employee or agent of the Board of Parole of the Department of Public Safety and Corrections to the extent that the employee or agent is authorized to access records containing HIV test results in order to implement the functions, powers, and duties with respect to the individual patient of the Board of Parole, Department of Public Safety and Corrections.

- An employee or agent of the office of probation and parole of the Department of Public Safety and Corrections, Division of Correction Services, to the extent that the employee or agent is authorized to access records containing HIV test results in order to carry out the functions, powers, and duties with respect to patient of the office.

- A medical director of a local correctional facility, to the extent that the medical director is authorized to access records containing HIV test results in order to carry out the functions, powers, and duties with respect to the patient.

- An employee or agent of the Department of Public Safety and Corrections, to the extent that employee or agent is authorized to access records containing HIV test results in order to carry out the Department of Public Safety and Corrections functions, powers, and duties with respect to the patient.

- An employee or agent who is authorized by the Department of Social Services, Office of Rehabilitative Services, to access records containing HIV test results in order to carry out the Department of Social Services, Office of Rehabilitative Services functions, powers, and duties with respect to the protected patient.

- An insurer, insurance administrator, self-insured employer, self-insurance trust, or other person or entity responsible for paying or

> determining payment for medical services, to the extent necessary to secure payment for those services (*Id.* § 1300.14).

No person to whom confidential HIV test results have been disclosed under this statute shall disclose the information to another person except as authorized by the statute (*Id.*).

Louisiana Code of Evidence article 510 provides for a privilege for communications for treatment of health conditions, including a condition induced by alcohol, drugs, or other substances.

Louisiana Code of Evidence article 510 provides for a privilege for mental health information involving communications between psychotherapists and patients.

Under Louisiana Revised Statutes § 28:171, mental patients have a right to privacy:

> No patient in a treatment facility pursuant to this Chapter shall be deprived of any rights, benefits, or privileges guaranteed by law, the Constitution of the State of Louisiana, or the Constitution of the United States solely because of his status as a patient in a treatment facility. These rights, benefits, and privileges include, but are not limited to, civil service status; the right to vote; the right to privacy; rights relating to the granting, renewal, forfeiture, or denial of a license or permit for which the patient is otherwise eligible; and the right to enter contractual relationships and to manage property [*Id.* § 28:171(A)].

Maine

Maine has a comprehensive statute covering AIDS testing, Maine Revised Statutes Title 5, §§ 19201-19208, which provides that no person, upon penalty of termination of employment or civil liability including damages and a fine of up to $1,000 for a negligent violation and $5,000 for an intentional violation, may disclose the results of an HIV test, except:

- To the subject of the test.
- To the subject's designated healthcare provider, who may only further disclose the information to other healthcare providers providing direct care to the subject.
- To others the subject has designated in writing.
- To healthcare providers who process donated human body parts to ensure medical acceptability of the gift.
- To certain research facilities if the subject's identity is kept confidential.

- To an anonymous testing site.

- To other agencies responsible for the treatment or care of the subject, including the Department of Corrections, the Department of Human Services, and the Department of Mental Health and Mental Retardation.

- To the Bureau of Health.

- As part of the medical record when disclosure has been authorized by the subject.

- Pursuant to court ordered disclosure.

Healthcare providers with patient records containing HIV infection status must have a written policy providing for confidentiality that requires, at a minimum, termination of employment for any employee who violates the confidentiality policy.

No medical record containing any test results may be disclosed in any proceeding without the patient's consent except in the following six cases:

- Proceedings under the communicable disease laws.

- Proceedings under the Adult Protective Services Act.

- Proceedings under child protection laws.

- Proceedings under mental health laws.

- Pursuant to a court order on a showing of good cause.

- For utilization review.

A patient may refuse to disclose and may prevent any person—including a physician, psychotherapist, or other persons participating in the patient's care—from disclosing confidential communications made for the purpose of diagnosis or treatment of a physical, mental, or emotional condition, including alcohol or drug addiction [Maine Revised Statutes Title 16, § 357; *Id.* Title 22, §§ 815(1) & 4015; *Id.* Title 32, § 1092-A; *Id.* Title 24-A, § 4224]. The privilege does not exist, however, if relevant to an issue in proceedings to hospitalize the patient for mental illness, if the patient was examined by court order, or if the condition is an element of the claim or defense (*Id.* Title 24, § 2510; *Id.* Title 25, § 2415).

Maryland

Maryland Code § 18-206 makes confidential all infectious or contagious disease reports (*Id.* § 18-201), cancer reports (*Id.* § 18-203), laboratory examination reports (*Id.* § 18-205), and sentinel birth defects reports (*Id.* § 18-206). Section 18-207(d) makes confidential required monthly reports of directors of medical laboratories concerning the identity of anyone tested for HIV.

Section 8-601 provides for confidentiality of alcohol and drug abuse information and specifies that the federal regulations govern disclosure and use of such records.

Sections 7-610 through 7-612 make confidential all developmental disability information.

Massachusetts

Chapter 111, section 119, makes records pertaining to venereal diseases confidential, as are records of HLTV-III tests (*Id.* chapter 111, § 70F).

The administrator of each alcoholism facility must keep records of treatment afforded patients confidential (*Id.* chapter 111B, § 11), as must administrators of drug rehabilitation facilities (*Id.* chapter 111E, § 18). The latter statute adds that disclosure may be made in accordance with the federal Drug Abuse Office and Treatment Act and 21 U.S.C. § 1175.

Any communication between an allied mental health or human services professional and a client is confidential (Massachusetts General Laws Chapter 112, § 172).

Chapter 175, § 108E, provides for confidentiality of insureds receiving mental health care. Similar rules exist with regard to mental health patients who are subscribers of medical service corporations in chapter 176B, § 20; those of nonprofit hospital service corporations in chapter 176A, § 14B; and those of health maintenance organizations in chapter 176G, § 4B.

Chapter 233, § 20B, establishes a patient-psychotherapist privilege.

Under Massachusetts General Laws Chapter 111, § 204, except as otherwise provided in the following, the proceedings, reports, and records of a medical peer review committee are confidential and are not subject to subpoena or discovery, or introduced into evidence, in any judicial or administrative proceeding, except proceedings held by the boards of registration in medicine, social work, or psychology.

Documents, incident reports, or records otherwise available from original sources are immune from subpoena, discovery, or use in any such judicial or administrative proceeding merely because they were presented to such committee in connection with its proceedings. Nor shall the proceedings, reports, findings, and records of a medical peer review committee be immune from subpoena, discovery, or use as evidence in any proceeding against a member of such committee to establish a cause of action pursuant to chapter 231, § 85N (damages as a result of acts within the scope of one's committee duties); provided, however, that in no event shall the identity of any person furnishing information or opinions to the committee be disclosed without the permission of such person. Nor shall the provisions of this section apply to any investigation or administrative proceeding conducted by the boards of registration in medicine, social work, or psychology (*Id.*).

Michigan

Michigan Compiled Laws § 333.5114a, governing HIV testing, provides that such information is exempt from disclosure under the Freedom of Information Act.

Section 333.5111 requires the Department of Health to promulgate rules to provide for the confidentially of reports, records, and data pertaining to research, among others, associated with communicable diseases or infections. Reports, records, and data pertaining to testing, care, treatment, reporting, and research associated with serious communicable diseases or HIV infection, acquired immunodeficiency syndrome (AIDS), and acquired immunodeficiency syndrome-related complex are confidential and may be released only as provided in the statute (*Id.* § 333.5131). AIDS information may be released to the Department of Public Health, a local health department, or other healthcare provider for one or more of the following reasons:

- To protect the health of an individual.

- To prevent further transmission of HIV.

- To diagnose and care for a patient [*Id.* § 333.5131(5)(a)].

Under Michigan Compiled Laws § 333.6111, records of the identity, diagnosis, prognosis, and treatment of an individual maintained in connection with the performance of a licensed substance-abuse treatment and rehabilitation service are confidential. Section 333.6113 specifies the circumstances under which a provider may disclose such a patient's record without consent.

Information in the records of recipients of mental health services and other information acquired in the course of providing mental health services to a recipient is confidential, and a facility may only disclose it under the circumstances outlined in Michigan Compiled Laws § 330.1748. When a facility discloses such information, the identity of the person to whom it pertains must be protected and may not be disclosed unless it is germane to the authorized purpose for which disclosure is sought.

Minnesota

Minnesota Statutes § 144.054 permits the health commissioner to subpoena privileged medical information of patients who may have been exposed to the human immunodeficiency virus (HIV) or hepatitis B virus (HBV) by a licensed dental hygienist, dentist, physician, nurse, podiatrist, a registered dental assistant, or a physician's assistant who is infected with such viruses when the commissioner has determined that it may be necessary to notify those patients that they may have been exposed to HIV or HBV.

Minnesota Regulation 4605.7702 requires confidentiality of venereal disease information.

Records of treatment for alcohol and drug abuse are confidential (*Id.* § 254A.09), as are records concerning drug and alcohol testing of employees (*Id.* § 181.954).

Revealing a communication from or relating to a mental health patient is prohibited conduct for mental health practitioners (*Id.* § 148B.68).

Mississippi

Testing and/or treatment for a sexually transmitted disease shall be kept in strict confidence (*Id.* § 41-23-30).

The registration and other records of services by alcoholism and alcohol abuse prevention, control, and treatment facilities are confidential, and the information that has been entered in them is privileged (*Id.* § 41-30-33).

Mississippi Code § 41-21-97 provides for confidentiality of records of patients who have been civilly committed.

Missouri

AIDS information and records held by any person, agency, department, or political subdivision of the state are strictly confidential and shall not be disclosed, except as discussed in Chapter 10. The Department of Mental Health shall not report to the Department of Health the identity of any individual for whom HIV testing confirms HIV infection if such reporting is prohibited by federal confidentiality laws or regulations (*Id.* § 191.662).

Section 191.317 provides for confidentiality of all test results and personal information obtained from any individual tested under genetics and metabolic disease programs.

Records compiled, obtained, prepared, or maintained by a residential facility or day program operated, funded, or licensed by the Department of Mental Health are confidential (*Id.* § 630.140).

Montana

Montana Code § 50-16-1009 provides for confidentiality of the identity of
a subject of an HIV-related test or the results of a test in a manner that
permits identification of the subject of the test. A person who discloses or
compels another to disclose confidential healthcare information in violation
of this section is guilty of a misdemeanor punishable by a fine of $1,000 or
imprsonment for one year, or both.

The registration and other records of treatment facilities are confidential and privileged under Montana Code § 53-24-306. Information from
such records may not be published in a way that discloses patients' names
or other identifying information.

Montana Code Annotated § 53-20-161 provides for confidentiality of
records concerning developmentally disabled persons, as does section 53-
21-166 for records concerning mental illness.

Montana Code Annotated § 26-1-807 establishes a psychologist-client
privilege.

Nebraska

Section 71-511 makes confidential all information concerning any patient
or test results involving communicable diseases. Similarly, laboratory notifications involving contagious diseases (*Id.* § 71-502.04) and data of the
cancer registry (*Id.* § 81-647; Nebraska Administrative Rules and Regulations 174-5-008) are confidential.

Nebraska follows the federal rules concerning confidentiality of alcohol and drug abuse records.

A newly proposed statute, 1993 Nebraska LB 669, would prohibit the
disclosure of mental health information except in enumerated circumstances.

Nevada

Nevada Revised Statutes § 441A.220 provides for confidentiality of communicable disease information. All information of a personal nature about
any person provided by any other person reporting a case or suspected case
of a communicable disease, by any person who has a communicable disease, or as determined by investigation of the health authority, is confidential medical information and must not be disclosed to any person under any
circumstances, including pursuant to any subpoena, search warrant, or discovery proceeding, except as follows:

- For statistical purposes, provided that the identity of the person is
  not discernible from the information disclosed.

- In a prosecution for a violation of the communicable disease laws.

- In a proceeding for an injunction brought pursuant to this chapter.

- In reporting the actual or suspected abuse or neglect of a child or elderly person.

- To any person who has a medical need to know the information for his or her own protection or for the well-being of a patient or dependent person, as determined by the health authority in accordance with regulations of the board.

- If the person who is the subject of the information consents in writing to the disclosure.

- Pursuant to the statute governing testing of sexual offenders for HIV.

- If the disclosure is made to the Welfare Division of the Department of Human Resources and the person about whom the disclosure is made has been diagnosed as having acquired immunodeficiency syndrome or an illness related to the human immunodeficiency virus and is a recipient of or an applicant for assistance to the medically indigent.

- To a firefighter, police officer, or person providing emergency medical services if the board has determined that the information relates to a communicable disease significantly related to that occupation.

- If the disclosure is authorized or required by specific statute.

Persons applying for or receiving treatment for alcohol or drug abuse have a right to confidentiality concerning any information relating thereto (*Id.* § 458.055).

The clinical record of a person hospitalized for mental illness is not a public record, and no part of it may be released, except as authorized by *Id.* § 433A.360.

New Hampshire

No one may disclose the identity of a person tested for the human immunodeficiency virus (New Hampshire Revised Statute Annotated § 141-F:8). Under New Hampshire law, all records and other information relating to persons testing for this virus shall be maintained as confidential and protected from inadvertent or unwarranted intrusion [New Hampshire Revised Statute Annotated § 141-F:8(I) & (II)]. Such information may be released, however, upon request if the patient has given written authorization or to other healthcare providers when necessary to protect the health of the patient tested. Anyone who purposely violates these confidentiality requirements and thereby discloses the identity of a person infected by the HIV virus is liable for actual damages, court costs, and attorney's fees, plus a civil penalty of up to $5,000 for such disclosure (*Id.* § 141-F:10) and guilty of a misdemeanor (*Id.* § 141-F:11).

A report provided to the director that identifies a specific individual as having a communicable disease may only be released to persons demonstrating a need that is essential to health-related research. Any release of information must be conditioned upon the personal identities remaining confidential. The physician-patient privilege does not apply to communicable disease information (*Id.* § 141-C:7).

Healthcare providers may not disclose the identity of an individual who was reported to the cancer registry as having cancer, except to persons demonstrating a need that is essential to health-related research. The release must be conditioned upon the personal identities of these cancer patients remaining confidential. The physician patient-privilege does not apply to reports to the cancer registry (*Id.* § 141-B:9).

Similarly, reports of critical health problems or other data that discloses the identity of such persons' problems may be made available only to persons who demonstrate a need for the material for health-related research. The physician-patient privilege does not apply to such reports (*Id.* § 141-A:5).

No reports or records or the information contained therein on any client of an alcohol or drug-abuse treatment facility is discoverable by the state in any criminal prosecution. No one may use such records for other than rehabilitation, research, statistical, or medical purposes, except upon the written consent of the person examined or treated (*Id.* § 172:8-a).

Any person who willfully discloses confidential information concerning a client in the mental health services system obtained as a result of auditing and monitoring activities is guilty of a violation of the rules governing the state mental health services system (*Id.* § 135-C:5).

Section 135-C:63-a provides for confidentiality for quality control assurance information of a community mental health program.

Communications between persons certified under the mental health practice laws and their clients are privileged (*Id.* § 330-A:19).

New Jersey

New Jersey Revised Statutes § 26:5C-5 provides for confidentiality of AIDS and HIV infection information. Healthcare providers may not disclose the content of records concerning diagnosed cases of AIDS or HIV infections unless the subject of the record, or his or her authorized representative if the patient is incompetent or deceased, has given prior written informed consent. If the prior written consent has not been obtained, the records can be disclosed only under the following conditions:

- To qualified personnel for the purpose of conducting scientific research under an approved protocol, but the person who is the subject of the record may not be identified in any report and research personnel may not disclose the patient's identity.

- To qualified personnel for the purpose of conducting management audits, financial audits, or program evaluations, but such personnel shall not identify the person who is the subject of the record in any report or otherwise disclose the patient's identity. The facility may not release identifying information to audit personnel unless it is vital to the audit or evaluation.

- To qualified personnel involved in medical education or in diagnosis or treatment of the person who is the subject of the record. Disclosure is limited to personnel who are directly involved in medical education or treatment of the patient.

- To the Department of Health as required by state or federal law.

- As permitted by rules and regulations adopted by the Commissioner of Health for purposes of disease prevention and control.

- In all other instances authorized by state or federal law (New Jersey Revised Statutes § 26:5C-8).

New Jersey also permits disclosure of such information pursuant to a court order conditioned on a showing of good cause (*Id.* § 26:5C-9). However, any person to whom such a record is disclosed must hold it as confidential and may not release it unless one of the conditions of the statute is met. A patient who is aggrieved as a result of a violation of this confidentiality statute may recover actual damages, reasonable attorney's fees, and costs. If the violation was reckless or intentionally malicious, the patient may recover punitive damages (*Id.* § 26:5C-14).

New Jersey follows the federal rules concerning privileged communications in drug or alcohol programs. *See* New Jersey Statutes § 2A:62A-17.

New Jersey Statute § 2A:62A-16 authorizes the disclosure of otherwise-confidential mental health information when necessary to warn potential victims of mental health patients.

New Mexico

Under the Human Immunodeficiency Virus Test Act, New Mexico Statute Annotated § 24-2B-6, no one may disclose the identity of any person and the tests results other than to:

- The subject of the test, the subject's legally authorized guardian or custodian, and any person designated, in a legally effective release, executed by the subject.

- An authorized agent, a credentialed or privileged physician, or an employee of a health facility or healthcare provider if the facility or provider itself is authorized to obtain the test results, the agent or employee provides patient care or handles or processes specimens of bodily fluids or tissues, and the agent or employee has a need to know such information.

- A health facility or healthcare provider that processes, procures, distributes, or uses:

  - Human body parts from deceased persons with respect to medical information regarding that person.

  - Semen that was provided prior to the effective date of the Human Immunodeficiency Virus Test Act for purposes of artificial insemination.

  - Bood or blood products for transfusion or injection.

  - Human body parts for transplant with respect to medical information regarding the donor recipient.

- Health facility staff committees or accreditation or oversight review organizations that are conducting program monitoring, evaluation or service (so long as any identity remains confidential).

- For purposes of application or reapplication for insurance coverage, an insurer or reinsurer upon whose request the test is performed [*Id.* § 24-2B-6(A)-(F), (H)].

Disclosure under this act must be accompanied by a written statement that includes the following or similar language:

This information has been disclosed to you from records whose confidentiality is protected by state law. State law prohibits you from making any further disclosure of such information without the specific written consent of the person to whom such information pertains, or as otherwise permitted by state law [*Id.* § 24-2B-7; *see also* Health Care Financial Management Association, *New Mexico Hospital Association Legal Handbook*, chapter 3, ¶ E (4) at 55-56 (rev. ed. 1991)].

New Mexico Statutes Annotated § 26-2-12 prohibits disclosure of the record of a resident of the state who voluntarily submits for treatment for alcoholism except on court order. Section 26-2-14 makes records on drug abuse treatment confidential.

New Mexico requires authorization by the patient for release of any information relating to a mental disorder or developmental disability from which a person who is well acquainted with the patient might recognize the patient, unless:

- The recipient of the information is a mental health or developmental disabilities professional working with the patient when access to such information is required for the treatment.

- Disclosure is necessary to protect against a clear and substantial risk of death or serious injury.

- In the case of a minor, the disclosure to a parent or guardian is essential for the minor's treatment.

- The disclosure is to an insurer who is contractually obligated to pay expenses for the patient's treatment (*Id.* § 43-1-19).

New York

New York Public Health Law § 2782 provides for confidentiality of HIV-related information, and § 2306 makes information concerning sexually transmissible diseases confidential. HIV and AIDS-related information is confidential and may not be disclosed except to:

- Protected individuals, or when such individual lacks capacity to consent, a person authorized pursuant to law to consent to health care for the individual.

- Any person to whom disclosure is authorized pursuant to a release of confidential HIV-related information.

- Agents or employees of a health facility or healthcare provider if (1) the agent or employee is permitted to access medical records; (2) the health facility or healthcare provider itself is authorized to obtain the HIV-related information; and (3) the agent or employee provides health care to the protected individual, or maintains or processes medical records for billing or reimbursement.

- Healthcare providers or health facilities when knowledge of the HIV-related information is necessary to provide appropriate care or treatment to the protected individual or child of the individual.

- Health facilities or healthcare providers, in relation to the procurement, processing, distributing, or use of a human body or body part including organs, tissues, eyes, bones, arteries, blood, semen, or other body fluids, for use in medical education, research, therapy, or for transplantation to individuals.

- Federal, state, county, or local health officers when such disclosure is mandated by federal or state law.

- Authorized agencies in connection with foster care or adoption of child.

- Insurance institutions or other third-party reimbursers or their agents to the extent necessary to reimburse healthcare providers for health services; provided that, where necessary, an otherwise appropriate authorization for such disclosure has been secured by the provider.

- Any person to whom disclosure is ordered by a court of competent jurisdiction.

- Employees or agents of the division of parole under certain circumstances.

- Employees or agents of the division of probation under certain circumstances.

- Medical directors of a local correctional facility under certain circumstances.

- Employees or agents or commissions of correction under certain circumstances.

- Law guardians, appointed to represent a minor pursuant to the social services law or the family court act, with respect to confidential HIV-related information relating to the minor and for the purpose of representing the minor. If the minor has capacity to consent, the law guardian may not redisclose the information without the minor's permission. If the minor does not have such capacity, the guardian may redisclose information for the sole purpose of representing the minor (*Id.* § 2782).

No person to whom confidential HIV-related information has been disclosed may disclose it to another person except as authorized by this statue (*Id.*).

A physician may disclose confidential HIV-related information under the following conditions:

- Disclosure is made to a contact or to a public health officer for the purpose of making the disclosure to said contact.

- The physician reasonably believes disclosure is medically appropriate and there is a significant risk of infection to the contact.

- The physician has counseled the protected individual regarding the need to notify the contact, and the physician reasonably believes the protected individual will not inform the contact.

- The physician has informed the protected individual of his or her intent to make such disclosure to a contact and has given the protected individual the opportunity to express a preference whether the physician should make the disclosure directly or to a public health officer [*Id.* § 2782(4)(a)].

A physician may also, upon the consent of a parent or guardian, disclose confidential HIV-related information to a health officer for the purpose of reviewing the medical history of a child to determine the fitness of the child to attend school (*Id.*).

The physician may also disclose such information to a person authorized to consent to health care for a protected individual when the physician reasonably believes that (1) disclosure is medically necessary in order to provide timely care and treatment for the protected individual; and (2) after appropriate counseling about the need for such disclosure the protected individual will not inform a person authorized by law to consent to health care. However, the physician shall not make such a disclosure if it would not be in the best interest of the protected individual or he or she is authorized by law to consent to such care and treatment [*Id.* § 2782(4)(e)].

Whenever anyone discloses confidential HIV-related information, except to the individual or the person authorized to consent to health care, the disclosure will be accompanied by a statement:

> This information has been disclosed to you from confidential records which are protected by state law. State law prohibits you from making any further disclosure of this information without the specific written consent of the person to whom it pertains, or as otherwise provided by law. Any unauthorized further disclosure in violation of state law may result in a fine or jail sentence or both. A general authorization for the release of medical or other information is NOT sufficient authorization for further disclosure [*Id.* § 2782(5)(a)].

All records of the identity, diagnosis, prognosis, or treatment in connection with a person's receipt of substance abuse services is confidential and may be released only in accordance with state and federal law (New York Consolidated Laws Service Mental Hygiene § 21.05).

New York Mental Hygiene Law § 33.13 provides for confidentiality of clinical records of clients or patients of facilities licensed or operated by the office of mental health or the office of mental retardation and developmental disabilities and contains detailed guidance on disclosure.

North Carolina

North Carolina law prohibits disclosure of records of cancer patients (North Carolina General Statute § 130A-212) and the records of persons identified as having the AIDS virus or other communicable or reportable diseases (*Id.* § 130A-143). All information and records that identify a person who has AIDS virus infection or who has or may have a reportable disease or condition must be strictly confidential. This information shall not be released or made public except under the following circumstances:

- Release is made of specific medical or epidemiological information for statistical purposes in a way that no person can be identified.
- Release is made of all or part of the medical record with the written consent of the person or persons identified or their guardians.
- Release is made to healthcare personnel providing medical care to the patient.
- Release is necessary to protect the public health and is made as provided by the commission in its rules regarding control measures for communicable diseases and conditions.
- Release is made pursuant to other provisions of this article.
- Release is made pursuant to subpoena or court order (*Id.*).
- Release is made by a health department to a court or law enforcement officer.
- Release is made by a health department to another public health agency to prevent or control the spread of a communicable disease.
- Release is made by the Department of Health for bona fide research purposes.
- Release is for communicable disease control.
- Release is otherwise authorized by law.

North Carolina follows the federal laws concerning alcohol and drug abuse record confidentiality. *See* North Carolina General Statutes § 8-44.1.

The Mental Health, Developmental Disabilities, and Substance Abuse Act (*Id.* § 122C-55). specifies confidentiality requirements for mental health, developmental disabilities, and substance abuse patients.

North Dakota

North Dakota requires healthcare providers, blood banks, blood centers, and plasma centers that obtain or test specimens of body fluids for HIV antibody to maintain records of consent to testing and the result of the tests (North Dakota Century Code § 23-07.5.) Such information is confidential (*Id.* § 23.07.5-05) and may only be released to:

- The subject of the test, which in the case of a minor is the parent or legal guardian or custodian of the subject, and in the case of an incapacitated person is the legal guardian of the subject. In the event the subject is in a foster home or to be adopted, the parent, legal guardian, or custodian may disclose the results to the foster parents or potential adoptive parents.

- The test subject's healthcare provider, including those instances in which a healthcare provider provides emergency care to the subject.

- An agent or employee of the test subject's healthcare provider who provides patient care or handles or processes specimens of body fluids or tissues.

- A blood bank, blood center, or plasma center that subjects a person to a test for any of the following purposes:

  - Determining the medical acceptability of blood or plasma secured from the test subject.

  - Notifying the test subject of the test results.

  - Investigating HIV infections in blood or plasma.

- A healthcare provider who procures, processes, distributes, or uses a donated human body party for the purpose of ensuring the medical acceptability of the gift for the purpose intended.

- The state health officer or his or her designee, for the purpose of providing epidemiologic surveillance or investigation or control of communicable disease.

- An embalmer.

- A healthcare facility staff committee or accreditation or health-care services review organization for the purposes of conducting program monitoring and evaluation and healthcare services reviews.
- A person who conducts research, if the researcher:
  - Is affiliated with the test subject's healthcare provider.
  - Has obtained permission to perform the research from an institutional review board.
  - Provides written assurance to the person disclosing the test results that the information requested is only for the purpose for which it is provided to the research, the information will not be released to a person not connected with the study, and the final research product will not reveal information that may identify the test subject unless the researcher has first received informed consent for disclosure from the test subject (*Id.*).

The test results may be disclosed under a lawful court order. In addition, the individual tested may authorize disclosure to any person (*Id.*).

North Dakota law provides for an addiction counselor-client privilege (*Id.* §§ 31-01-06.3 through 06.6). The privilege covers confidential communications made for the purpose of treating the client's physical, mental, or emotional condition, including alcohol or drug addiction, among the client, the client's counselor, and those participating in the diagnosis or treatment under the direction of the counselor (*Id.* § 31-01-06.4).

All documents, records, information, memoranda, reports, complaints, or written or nonwritten communication relating to an identified or identifiable person with developmental disabilities or mental illness are confidential and not subject to disclosure except in limited circumstances enumerated in North Dakota Century Code § 25-10.3-10.

Ohio

Ohio Revised Code § 3701.241 requires the health director to develop and administer a program for confidential and anonymous AIDS testing and a confidential partner notification system. Under Ohio Administrative Code 3701-3-08, communicable disease information is confidential.

Ohio Revised Code § 3793.12 makes communications confidential that are made by a person seeking aid in good faith for alcoholism or drug dependence, and § 3793.13 provides for confidentiality of records of drug abuse treatment programs. Ohio Administrative Code 3701-55-15(c) amplifies this guidance by noting that all information contained in records of alcohol inpatient/emergency care patient records is confidential, and the provider shall only disclose it to authorized persons.

All records of the Department of Mental Retardation and Developmental Disabilities—other than court journal entries or court docket entries, which directly or indirectly identify a resident or former resident of an institution for the mentally retarded or person whose institutionalization has been sought—are confidential and shall not be disclosed with limited exceptions (Ohio Revised Code § 5123.89). Reports of abuse of mentally retarded adults are not public records [*Id.* § 5123.61(j)]. Records of those hospitalized for mental illness are confidential and may only be disclosed as specified in the statute *(Id.* § 5122.31).

Oklahoma

Reports concerning venereal and other statutorily designated diseases are confidential [Oklahoma Statutes Title 63, § 1-502.2(A)] and may be released only under the following circumstances:

- Release is made upon court order.

- Release is made in writing, by or with the written consent of the person whose information is being kept confidential or with the written consent of the legal guardian or legal custodian of such person, or if such person is a minor, with the written consent of the parent or legal guardian of such minor.

- Release is necessary as determined by the state Department of Health to protect the health and well-being of the general public. Any such order for release by the department and any review of such order shall be in accordance with the procedures specified by the law. Only the initials of the person whose information is being kept confidential shall be on public record for such proceedings unless the order by the department specifies the release of the name of such person and such order is not appealed by such person or such order is upheld by the reviewing court.

- Release is made of medical or epidemiological information to those persons who have had risk exposure to communicable diseases [*Id.* (referring to section 1-502.1)].

- Release is made of medical or epidemiological information to health professionals, appropriate state agencies, or district courts to enforce the Oklahoma law and related rules and regulations concerning the control and treatment of communicable or venereal diseases.

- Release is made of specific medical or epidemiological information for statistical purposes in such a way that no person can be identified.

- Release is made of medical information among healthcare providers within a therapeutic environment for the purpose of diagnosis and treatment of the person whose information is released. This exception shall not authorize the release of confidential information by a state agency to a healthcare provider unless such release is otherwise authorized by this section (*Id.*).

Violation of the confidentiality requirements is a misdemeanor [*Id.* Title 63, § 1-502.2(D)] and makes the offender liable for any civil damages caused by the disclosure [*Id.* Title 63, § 1-502.2(E)].

Birth defects information (*Id.* Title 63, § 1-550.2) and tumor registry information (*Id.* Title 63, § 1-551.1) are confidential and may only be divulged under limited circumstances.

Under the Oklahoma Alcohol and Drug Abuse Services Act, all medical records and communications between doctor and patient are privileged and confidential and will not be released to anyone not involved in the treatment programs without a written release from the patient or a court order. Such information must be kept in folders clearly marked "Confidential" (*Id.* Title 43A, § 3-422).

Except as specified in 43A Oklahoma Statutes § 1-109, all medical records between physicians or psychotherapists and patients are privileged and confidential. Such information is available only to persons or agencies actively engaged in treatment of the patient and treatment of a minor child of the patient, or in related administrative work.

Oregon

Oregon Revised Statutes § 433.045(3) states that no person shall disclose the identity of a person upon whom an HIV-related test was performed or the results of such a test in a manner that permits identification of the person unless he or she authorizes the disclosure or it is required by law.

The records of a patient at a drug or alcohol addiction treatment facility shall not be disclosed without the consent of the patient [*Id.* § 426.460(5)].

Oregon Revised Statutes § 430.763 provides for confidentiality of records of abuse reporting for the mentally ill or developmentally disabled.

Pennsylvania

Pennsylvania's Confidentiality of HIV-Related Information Act defines such information as "any information which is in the possession of a person who provides one or more health or social services or who obtains the information pursuant to a release of confidential HIV-related information and which concerns whether an individual has been the subject of an HIV-related test, or has HIV, HIV-related illness, or AIDS; or any information which identifies or reasonably could identify an individual as having one or more of these conditions, including information pertaining to the individual's contacts."

Section 7607 provides for the confidentiality of records. No person or employee, or agent of such person, who obtains confidential HIV-related information in the course of providing any health or social service or pursuant to a release of confidential HIV-related information under subsection (c) may disclose or be compelled to disclose the information, except to the following persons:

- The subject.
- The physician who ordered the test, or the physician's designee.
- Any person specifically designated in a written consent.
- An agent, employee, or medical staff member of a healthcare provider, when the healthcare provider has received confidential HIV-related information during the course of the subject's diagnosis or treatment by the healthcare provider, provided that the agent, employee, or medical staff member is involved in the medical care or treatment of the subject.
- A peer review organization or committee, a nationally recognized accrediting agency, or as otherwise provided by law, any federal or state government agency with oversight responsibilities for healthcare providers.
- Individual healthcare providers involved in the care of the subject with an HIV-related condition or a positive test, when knowledge of the condition or test result is necessary to provide emergency care or treatment appropriate to the individual, or healthcare providers consulted to determine diagnosis and treatment of the individual.
- An insurer, to the extent necessary to reimburse healthcare providers or to make any payment of a claim submitted pursuant to an insured's policy.

- The department of health and persons authorized to gather, transmit, or receive vital statistics.

- The department of health and local boards and departments of health for purposes of disease prevention and control.

- A person allowed access to the information by a court order issued pursuant to § 7608.

- A funeral director responsible for the acceptance and preparation of the deceased subject.

- Employees of county mental health/mental retardation agencies, county children and youth agencies, county juvenile probation departments, county or state facilities for delinquent youth, and contracted residential providers of the previously named entities receiving or contemplating residential placement of the subject, who:

  - Generally are authorized to receive medical information.

  - Are responsible for ensuring that the subject receives appropriate health care.

  - Have a need to know the HIV-related information in order to ensure such care is provided.

Nothing in this statute requires the segregation of confidential HIV-related information from a subject's medical record.

No person to whom confidential HIV-related information has been disclosed under this act may disclose that information to another person, except as authorized by this act.

An institutional healthcare provider that has access to or maintains individually identifying confidential HIV-related information shall establish written procedures for confidentiality and disclosure of the records that are in accordance with the provisions of this act.

71 Pennsylvania Consolidated Statutes § 1690.108 provides for confidentiality of records of alcohol and drug abuse patients. 55 Pennsylvania Code § 5100.37 adds that whenever information in a patient's records relates to drug or alcohol abuse or dependency, those records are subject to the 71 Pennsylvania Consolidated Statutes § 1690.108, previously described.

General and special hospitals' psychiatric services must ensure the confidentiality of each patient receiving treatment (28 Pennsylvania Code § 155.8).

Records of persons seeking, receiving, or having received mental health services are confidential. Providers must inform each client/patient of the specific limits on confidentiality that affect his or her treatment. The custodian of such records must exercise control over the release of information contained therein. This regulation adds that when information and observations regarding clients or patients are not made a part of the record, there remains a duty and obligation for the staff to respect the patient's privacy and confidentiality by acting ethically and responsibly in using or discussing such information (55 Pa. Code § 5100.310). *Id.* §§ 5100.32, .33, .34, and .35 contain guidelines for nonconsensual release of such information, patient access, consent for release to third parties, and to the courts, respectively.

Rhode Island

Rhode Island general laws provide that no person may disclose the results of another person's AIDS test without the prior written consent of that individual—or, in the case of a minor, of the minor's parent, guardian, or agent—on a form that specifically states that the AIDS test result may be released (Rhode Island General Law § 23-6-17). However, a licensed laboratory or healthcare facility that performs AIDS tests may release the results to a physician and to the director of the Department of Health.

A physician may disclose the test results to other health professionals involved in the care of a person who tests positive for the AIDS virus and to persons who are in close contact with or exposed to bodily fluids of a person who tests positive for AIDS if there is, in the physician's opinion, a clear and present danger of transmission of the virus to the third party [*Id.* § 23-6-17(a) and (b)].

The registration and other records of alcoholism treatment facilities are confidential and privileged to the patient (*Id.* § 40.1-4-13).

General Laws of Rhode Island § 40.1-5-18 provide for confidentiality of mental health information received by the mental health advocate, his or her assistants, and every employee of his or her office.

Id. § 40.1-5-26 governs disclosure of confidential mental health information and records.

The fact of admission to a community residence and all information and records compiled, obtained, or maintained in the course of providing mental health or retardation services are confidential (*Id.* § 40.1-24.5-11).

South Carolina

All information and records held by the Department of Health and Environmental Control and its agents relating to a known or suspected case of a sexually transmitted disease are strictly confidential. The information must not be released or made public, upon subpoena or otherwise, except under the following circumstances:

- Release is made of medical or epidemiological information for statistical purposes in a manner that no individual person can be identified.

- Release is made of medical or epidemiological information with the consent of all persons identified in the information released.

- Release is made of medical or epidemiological information to the extent necessary to enforce the provisions of this chapter and related regulations concerning the control and treatment of a sexually transmitted disease.

- Release is made of medical or epidemiological information to medical personnel to the extent necessary to protect the health or life of any person.

- In cases involving a minor, the name of the minor and medical information concerning the minor must be reported to appropriate agents if a report is required by the Child Protection Act of 1977. No further information is required to be released by the department. If a minor has acquired immunodeficiency syndrome (AIDS) or is infected with human immunodeficiency virus (HIV) and is attending the public schools, the superintendent of the school district and the nurse or other health professional assigned to the school that the minor attends must be notified (South Carolina Code § 44-29-135).

South Carolina Code § 44-52-190 makes records of alcohol and drug abuse commitment confidential.

South Carolina Code § 44-20-340 makes confidential the records of mentally retarded or developmentally disabled patients. Section 44-23-1090 reiterates confidentiality of information about patients who are mentally ill or retarded. Regulation 61-13, § 501 states that medical records of residents of intermediate care facilities' mental retardation are confidential.

South Dakota

South Dakota Codified Laws § 34-22-12.1 provides for confidentiality of reports of communicable diseases. Such reports are strictly confidential medical information. Such reports may not be released, shared with any agency or institution, or made public upon subpoena, search warrant, discovery proceedings, or otherwise. The reports are not admissible as evidence in any action of any kind in any court or before any tribunal, board, agency, or person, except that release of medical or epidemiological information may be made or authorized by the Department of Health under any of the following circumstances:

- For statistical purposes in such a manner that no person can be identified.
- With the written consent of the person identified in the information released.
- To the extent necessary to enforce the provisions of the law concerning the prevention, treatment, control, and investigation of communicable diseases.
- To the extent necessary to protect the health or life of a named person.

Test results of HIV testing of suspects of sexual assault are confidential under *Id.* § 23A-35B-5.

South Dakota Codified Laws Annotated § 34-20A-91 requires information used for research into the causes and treatment of alcohol abuse to be kept confidential and not published in a way that discloses patients' names or other identifying information.

Rule 503 of the South Dakota Rules of Evidence establishes a psychotherapist-patient privilege (South Dakota Codified Laws § 19-13-7).

Information in a person's record and other information acquired in the course of providing mental health services to a person is confidential and may only be disclosed as specified in the statutes and in conformity with federal law (*Id.* § 27A-12-26).

Tennessee

All records and information held by the Department of Health and Environment or a local health department relating to known or suspected cases of sexually transmitted disease are confidential and may only be released in the limited circumstances (*Id.* § 68-10-113). Such information shall not be released or made public upon subpoena, court order, discovery, search warrant, or otherwise, except that release may be made under the following circumstances:

- Release is made of medical or epidemiological information to medical personnel, appropriate state agencies, or county and district courts to enforce the provisions of this chapter and related regulations governing the control and treatment of sexually transmitted diseases.
- In a case involving a minor not more than 13 years of age, only the name, age, address, and sexually transmitted disease treated shall be

reported to appropriate agents as required by the Tennessee Child Abuse Law. No other information shall be released. If the information to be disclosed is required in a court proceeding involving child abuse, the information shall be disclosed *in camera.*

- Release is made during a legal proceeding when ordered by a trial court judge, designated by section 16-2-502, through an order explicitly finding each of the following:

  - The information sought is material, relevant, and reasonably calculated to be admissible evidence during the legal proceeding.

  - The probative value of the evidence outweighs the individual's and the public's interests in maintaining its confidentiality.

  - The merits of the litigation cannot be fairly resolved without the disclosure.

  - The evidence is necessary to avoid substantial injustice to the party seeking it, and either the disclosure will result in no significant harm to the person examined or treated, or it would be substantially unfair as between the requesting party and the person examined or treated not to require the disclosure (*Id.*).

However, before making such findings, the trial court judge may examine the information *in camera* and may order the information placed under seal [*Id.* § 68-10-113(6)(B)].

Under § 68-1-108, the insurance commission may release health insurance entities' report of UB-82 claims data but must keep any individual medical information confidential.

All applications, certificates, records, reports, and all legal documents, petitions, and records made by providers or information received under the laws governing the mentally ill and mentally retarded persons that directly or indirectly identify a patient or resident or former patient or resident are confidential and may only be disclosed under the limited circumstances specified in Tennessee Code § 33-3-104.

Texas

Texas Health and Safety Code Annotated § 81.046 provides for confidentiality of reports, records, and information relating to communicable diseases.

A test result for AIDS and related disorders is confidential and a person who knows of a test result may not disclose the test result except as provided under the statute [Texas Health & Safety Code Annotated § 81.103(a)]. The test result may be disclosed to the following:

- Department of Health.
- Local health authority if reporting is required by the law, governing communicable diseases.
- Centers for Disease Control if reporting is required by federal law or regulation.
- Physician or other person authorized by law who ordered the test.
- Physicians, nurses, or other health personnel who have a legitimate need to know the test results in order to provide for their protection and to provide for the patient's health and welfare.
- Persons tested or persons legally authorized to consent to the test on the patient's behalf.
- Spouse of the person tested if the person tests positive for AIDS or HIV infection, antibodies to HIV, or infection with any other probable causative agent of AIDS and if the physician who ordered the test makes the notification.
- Victims of sexual offenses [Texas Code Criminal Procedure Annotated article 21.31(a) (qualifying victims are listed in this article)] if the person tested allegedly committed the offense and the test was required under that article [*Id.*; Texas Health & Safety Code Annotated § 81.103(b)].

A blood bank may report positive blood test results indicating the name of a donor with possible infectious disease to other blood banks if it does not disclose the infectious disease the donor has or is suspected of having. The bank may report blood test results to hospitals where the blood was transfused, to the physician who transfused it, and to the recipient. It may disclose the results for statistical purposes. Such a report may not disclose the name of the donor or the person tested or any information that could result in the disclosure of the donor's or person's name, including an address, social security number, designated recipient, or replacement information [*Id.* § 81.103(g)].

A healthcare facility employee whose job requires him or her to deal with permanent medical records may view test results in the performance of his or her duties under reasonable healthcare facility practices [*Id.* § 81.103(i)]. However, anyone who releases or discloses a test result in violation of this section commits a misdemeanor when he or she, with criminal negligence, releases or discloses a test result or other information [*Id.* § 81.103(j)].

Hospital Licensing Standards permit disclosure of medical record information maintained by special care facilities for reporting of communicable disease information (Texas Department of Health, Hospital Licensing Standards chapter 12, § 8.7.3.1).

Communications between a patient or client and his or her physician for the purpose of diagnosis, evaluation, or treatment of alcoholism and drug abuse, described in Texas Code of Criminal Procedure article 38.101, are confidential and will not be disclosed except in limited circumstances.

Sections 533.010 and 595.001 provide for confidentiality of records of the identity, diagnosis, evaluation, or treatment of any person maintained in connection with the performance of any program or activity relating to mental retardation. Communications between a patient or client and his or her physician for the purpose of diagnosis, evaluation, or treatment of any mental or emotional disorder, including sex offenders, which are Texas Revised Civil Statute article 4413(51), are confidential and will not be disclosed except in limited circumstances.

Utah

Section 26-25a-101 provides for confidentiality of information regarding communicable or reportable diseases.

All reports or test results received by an employer through a drug or alcohol testing program are confidential (Utah Code § 34-38-13).

Mental retardation facilities shall keep confidential all information contained in clients' records as well as protect records against access by unauthorized individuals (*Id.* at 432-152-4.201 and 432-15-4.203).

Vermont

Vermont law makes tuberculosis reports (*Id.* Title 18, § 1041) and venereal disease reports confidential (*Id.* Title 18, § 1099).

Title 12, section 1705(a), governing HIV-related testing information, provides that Vermont state courts shall not issue any orders requiring the disclosure of individually identifiable HIV-related testing or counseling information, unless such court finds that the person seeking the information has demonstrated a compelling need for it that cannot be accommodated by other means.

A mental health professional, among others, may not disclose any information acquired in attending a patient in a professional capacity, and which was necessary to enable the provider to act in that capacity (12 Vermont Statutes § 1612).

Virginia

Virginia Code Annotated § 32.1-36.1(A) states that results of test for HIV are confidential and may be released, among others, to:

- The subject of the test or his or her legally authorized representative.
- Any person designated in a release signed by the subject of the test or his or her legally authorized representative.
- The Department of Health.
- Healthcare providers for the purposes of consultation or providing care and treatment to the person who was the subject of the test.
- Any facility that procures, processes, distributes, or uses blood, other body fluids, tissues, or organs.
- Any person authorized by law to receive such information.
- The parents of the subject of the test if the subject is a minor.
- The spouse of the subject of the test.

A willful or grossly negligent unauthorized disclosure subjects the offender to a $5,000 civil penalty as well as to payment of actual damages or $100, whichever is greater [*Id.* § 32.1-36.1(B) and (C)].

Persons who are patients or residents in a hospital or other facility operated, funded, or licensed by the Department of Mental Health, Mental Retardation, and Substance Abuse Services must be assured of the confidentiality of their medical and mental records *(Id.* § 37.1-84.1).

Section 37.1-228 prohibits disclosure of mental health patient information by third party payers except under certain conditions.

Washington

Records of HIV antibody testing and testing or treatment records of sexually transmitted disease patients *(Id.* § 70.24.105) are confidential. No person may disclose or be compelled to disclose the identity of any person upon whom an HIV antibody test is performed or the results of such a test. Nor may any person disclose the result of a test for any other sexually transmitted disease when it is positive or disclose any information relating to diagnosis of or treatment for HIV infection or any other confirmed sexually transmitted disease [Washington Revised Code § 70.24.105(1)]. The following persons, however, may receive such information:

- The subject of the test or the subject's legal representative for healthcare decisions, except for such a representative of a minor child more than 14 years of age and otherwise competent.

- Any person who secures a specific release or test results or information executed by the subject or the subject's legal representative for healthcare decisions, except for such a representative of a minor child more than 14 years of age and otherwise competent.

- The state public health officer, a local public health officer, or the Centers for Disease Control in accordance with reporting requirements for a diagnosed case of a sexually transmitted disease.

- A health facility or healthcare provider that procures, processes, distributes, or uses:

  - A human body part, tissue, or blood from a deceased person with respect to medical information regarding that person.

  - Semen, including that provided prior to March 23, 1988, for the purpose of artificial insemination.

  - Blood specimens.

- Any state or local public health officer conducting an investigation [*Id.* § 70.24.105(2)(e) (referring to section 70.24.024)] to determine whether an infected person is engaging in conduct that endangers the public health, provided that such record was obtained by means of court order for HIV testing.

- A person allowed access to the record by a court order granted after application showing good cause.

- Persons who, because of their behavioral interaction with the infected individual, have been placed at risk for acquisition of a sexually transmitted disease, if the health officer or authorized representative believes that the exposed person was unaware that a risk of disease exposure existed and that the disclosure of the identity of the infected person is necessary.

- A law enforcement officer, firefighter, healthcare provider, healthcare facility staff person, or other person as defined by the board of health who requested a test of a person whose bodily fluids he or she has been substantially exposed to, if a state or local public health officer performs the test.

- Claims management personnel employed by or associated with an insurer, healthcare service contractor, health maintenance organization, self-funded health plan, state-administered healthcare claims payer, or any other payer of healthcare claims by which such disclosure is to be used solely for the prompt and accurate evaluation and payment of medical or related claims. Information released under this subsection must be confidential and may not be released or available to persons who are not involved in handling or determining medical claims payment.

- A department of social and health services worker, a child-placement agency worker, or a guardian *ad litem* who is responsible for making or reviewing placement or case-planning decisions or recommendations to the court regarding a child who is less than 14 years of age, has a sexually transmitted disease, and is in the custody of the Department of Social and Health Services or a licensed child-placement agency. This information may also be received by a person responsible for providing residential care for such a child when the Department of Social and Health Services or a licensed child-placement agency determines that it is necessary for the provision of child care services [*Id.* § 70.24.105(2)].

No person to whom the results of a test for a sexually transmitted disease have been disclosed may disclose the results to another except as authorized in the preceding [*Id.* § 70.24.105(3)]. Whenever disclosure is made—except to the subject or his or her representative for healthcare decisions, or among healthcare providers in order to provide healthcare services—the disclosure must be accompanied by a written statement:

This information has been disclosed to you from records whose confidentiality is protected by state law. State law prohibits you from making any further disclosure of it without the specific written consent of the person to whom it pertains, or as otherwise permitted by state law. A general authorization for the release of medical or other information is NOT sufficient for this purpose [*Id.* § 70.24.105(5)].

If the disclosure is oral, the discloser will provide the written notice just listed within 10 days (*Id.*).

Records of alcoholics and intoxicated persons are confidential (*Id.* § 70.96A.150).

Revised Code of Washington § 71.05.630 provides that treatment records of mental illness patients are confidential and may only be released under limited circumstances.

West Virginia

Section 16-3C-3 makes confidential the identity of a person upon whom an HIV-related test is performed or the results of such a test that permits identification of the subject of the test, disclosure permitted only in limited circumstances. No person may disclose or be compelled to disclose the identity of any person upon whom an HIV-related test is performed or the results of such a test in a manner that permits identification of the subject of the test [West Virginia Code § 16-3C-3(a)(1)-(7)], except, among others, to:

- The subject of the test.

- Any person who secures a specific release of test results executed by the subject.

- Funeral directors, authorized agents, or employees of a health facility or healthcare provider, if the funeral establishment, health facility, or provider itself is authorized to obtain the test results, if the agent or the employee provides patient care or handles or processes specimens of body fluids or tissues, and if the agent or employee has a need to know such information. The recipient must maintain the confidentiality of the information.

- Licensed medical personnel or appropriate healthcare personnel providing care to the subject of the test—when knowledge of the test results is necessary or useful to provide appropriate care or treatment, in an appropriate manner—provided that such personnel must maintain the confidentiality of such test results.

- Department of Health or Centers for Disease Control in accordance with reporting requirements for a diagnosed case of AIDS or a related condition.

- Health facilities or healthcare providers that procure, process, distribute, or use:

  - A human body part from a deceased person with respect to medical information about him or her.

  - Semen provided prior to September 1, 1988 for the purpose of artificial insemination.

  - Blood or blood products for transfusion or injection.

  - Human body parts for transplant with regard to medical information regarding the donor or recipient.

- Health facility staff committees or accreditation or oversight review organizations that are conducting program monitoring, program evaluation, or services reviews so long as any identity remains anonymous (*Id.*).

The statute also permits disclose to inform sex partners or contacts or persons who have shared needles that they may be at risk of having acquired the HIV infection, but the name or identity of the person whose test was positive is to remain confidential [*Id.* § 16-3C-3(b)].

Whenever anyone discloses information under this statute but does not fall within one of the exceptions just listed, that person must add a written statement:

This information has been disclosed to you from records whose confidentiality is protected by state law. State law prohibits you from making any further disclosure of the information without the specific written consent of the person to whom it pertains, or as otherwise permitted by law. A general authorization for the release of medical or other information is NOT sufficient for this purpose [*Id.* § 16-3C-3(c)].

Section 16-4A-3 makes confidential the laboratory reports of blood tests for syphilis of pregnant women.

West Virginia Code § 27-3-1 provides for confidentiality of communications and treatment of mentally ill patients, including the fact that a person is or has been a client or patient and provides limited circumstances under which confidential information may be disclosed.

Wisconsin

Section 254.07 makes confidential the reports, examinations, inspections, and all records concerning sexually transmitted diseases.

Results of tests for the presence of HIV or an HIV antibody may not be disclosed, without the subject's consent [Wisconsin Statute § 146.025(2)(a)(5m)], except to the following, among others:

- The subject of the test.
- Healthcare providers.
- Blood banks.
- State epidemiologist.
- Funeral directors.
- Healthcare facility staff committees or accreditation or healthcare services review organizations.
- Under court order.
- Researchers.
- Persons who renders aid to the victim of an accident if exposed thereby to the disease.
- A coroner.

- Sheriffs or jail keepers.
- Those who have had sexual contact with the subject or who shared intravenous drug use paraphernalia, if the person is deceased.

No person to whom such test results have been disclosed may disclose the results except under the same rules [*Id.* § 146.025(5)].

The healthcare provider, blood bank, or plasma center that obtains specimens to test for HIV must maintain a record of informed consent for testing or disclosure and maintain a record of the results [*Id.* § 146.025(4)]. Notwithstanding the confidentiality requirements, such persons may only report positive tests results for HIV or an antibody to:

- The state epidemiologist for the purpose of providing epidemiologic surveillance or investigation or control of communicable disease.
- Healthcare facilities staff committees or accreditation or healthcare services review organizations for the purposes of conducting program monitoring and evaluation and healthcare services reviews.
- Researchers, if the researcher is affiliated with a healthcare provider, has obtained permission to perform the research from an institutional review board, and provides written assurance to the person disclosing the tests results of the following. Use of the information is only for the purpose for which it is provided to the researcher; the information will not be released to a person not connected with the study; and the final research product will not reveal information that may identify the subject, unless the researcher has first received informed consent for disclosure from the subject [Wisconsin Statute § 146.025(5)(a), (8), and (10)].

The healthcare provider, blood bank, or plasma center that obtains specimens to test for HIV may report positive tests results for HIV or an antibody, when required by law, to:

- Sheriffs, jailers, or keepers of a prison, a jail, or a house of correction to permit the assigning of a private cell to a prisoner with a positive test result.
- Coroners, medical examiners, or appointed assistants, if the possible HIV-infected status is relevant to the cause of death of a death under direct investigation, or if the coroner, medical examiners, or appointed assistants are significantly exposed to a person whose death is under direct investigation, or a physician certifies in writing that such individuals have been significantly exposed and the certification accompanies the request for disclosure [*Id.* § 146.025(5)(a)(12) and (13)].

Violations of this statute can result in civil liability of up to $5,000 or a criminal penalty [*Id.* § 146.025(8) and (9)].

Records concerning individuals who have received services for mental illness, developmental disabilities, alcoholism, or drug dependence are confidential and may be released only pursuant to informed consent or as provided for by the statute [*Id.* 51.30(2)]. Similarly, section 51.45 provides for confidentiality of registration and treatment records of alcoholism treatment programs and facilities.

Wisconsin Administrative Code § HSS 92.03 establishes further rights to privacy for patients who received treatment for mental illness, developmental disability, and alcohol and drug abuse, except those provided by individual practitioners. Under HSS 92.03, records that in any way identify a patient are confidential and may be released only upon informed consent by the patient or:

- For management audits, financial audits, or program monitoring and evaluation.
- For billing or collection.
- For research.
- By court order.
- For progress determination and to determine adequacy of treatment.
- Within the department.
- In medical emergencies.
- To facilities receiving an involuntarily committed person.
- To correctional facilities or probation and parole agencies.
- To counsel, guardians ad litem, counsel for the interest of the public, and court-appointed examiners.
- To correctional officers of a change in status.
- Between a social services department and a community programs board.
- Between subunits of a human services department and between the human services department and contracted service providers.
- To law enforcement officers when necessary to return a patient on unauthorized absence from the facility.

Wyoming

Wyoming Statutes § 35-4-132, which requires the reporting of communicable diseases, provides that information and records relating to a known or suspected case of sexually transmitted disease that has been so reported, are confidential and except as otherwise required by law, shall not be disclosed unless the disclosure is:

- For statistical purposes, provided that the identity of the individual with the known or suspected case is protected.

- Necessary for the control and treatment of sexually transmitted diseases.

- Made with the written consent of the individual identified within the information or records.

- For notification of healthcare professionals and health care employees as necessary to protect life and health.

Similarly, reports of required tests for sexually transmitted diseases when bodily fluids may have been criminally transferred are confidential under § 7-1-109.

A counselor, social worker, or chemical dependency specialist may not disclose without consent of the client any communication made by the client in the course of professional practice (Wyoming Statutes § 33-38-109).

Wyoming Statutes § 33-27-103 provides for privileged communications between psychologists and their clients.

Conclusion

Federal and state laws provide for enhanced confidentiality protection for sexually transmitted/communicable disease information, alcohol and drug abuse information, and mental health/developmental disabilities information. Because these statutes often provide severe sanctions for improper disclosure of such sensitive information and the courts have enforced these statutes stringently, providers must ensure that they provide extra protection for such sensitive healthcare information.

Endnotes

1. *Doe v. Row,* No. 0369 (N.Y. App. Div., 4th Dept., May 28, 1993).

2. Joint Commission on Accreditation of Healthcare Organizations, *1994 Accreditation Manual for Hospitals* Standard IM.2.2.2.

3. Section 35-38-1-7 has been repealed.

5

Confidentiality of Research Information

Introduction

Most states allow medical staff access to patients' records for medical research. However, even when a researcher has such access, the patients who are the subject of the research retain their rights to confidentiality. Thus, most laws authorizing disclosure for research require researchers to delete all information that would identify the patient from any research reports unless the patient has consented to being identified.

Healthcare facilities should have written procedures documenting policy on use of records for research covering, for example, access for staff, nonphysician healthcare providers, and investigators; approval authority; and security controls.

Federal Laws

Alcohol and drug abuse programs must maintain confidentiality certificates to protect the privacy of research subjects. The retention period is not specified [29 CFR § 2a (1991)].

The Social Security Administration (SSA) and Health and Human Services (HHS) departments release information held by them for research and statistical studies. The Privacy Act, 5 U.S.C. § 522a (1988), allows disclosure of records held by these departments, but the records may not contain personal identifiers unless the identifiers are necessary for the research project and the department receives assurance from the requesting party that ensures the privacy of the individuals subject to the records. The departments will also release personal identifiers if the recipient guarantees the records safety and submits to on-site inspection of those safeguards [20 CFR § 401.325 (1991)].

HHS also has procedures to protect the privacy of research subjects in federally funded research studies [*Id.* (found at 45 CFR § 46.102 *et seq.* (1991)].

State Laws

Most states have laws authorizing release of medical information for research and requiring anonymity for the research subjects. However, even if a particular state does not have a statute governing disclosure for medical research, a provider may nonetheless do so if patients' identities are protected. Of course, the prudent course, regardless of whether the state has such a law, is to get the patient's consent for the necessary disclosure at the same time the research obtains the informed consent for the research.

Alabama

Alabama has no specific rules for research other than the general confidentiality provisions outlined for states generally.

Alaska

Providers may release patient records and information without consent for research projects authorized by the governing board, if provision is made to preserve anonymity in the reported results [Alaska Administrative Code title 7, § 13.130(b)(3)].

Arizona

Providers may release records to persons doing research or maintaining health statistics, provided the department establishes rules for the conduct of such research to ensure the anonymity of the patient [Arizona Revised Statutes § 36-509 (A)].

Arkansas

Under Arkansas Code Annotated § 20-9-304, all information, interviews, reports, statements, memoranda, or other data of the State Board of Health, Arkansas Medical Society, allied medical societies, or in-hospital staff committees of licensed hospitals, but not the original medical records of patients used in the course of medical studies for the purpose of reducing morbidity or mortality, shall be strictly confidential and shall be used only for medical research. Any authorized person, hospital, sanatorium, nursing home, rest home, or other organization may provide such information relating to the condition and treatment of any person to the entities just listed for use in the course of studies for the purpose of reducing morbidity or mortality without incurring liability for damages or other relief. However, in any event, the patient's identity is confidential and will not be released under any circumstances.

California

A provider may release medical information to researchers if the director of mental health or developmental disabilities designates by regulation a set of rules for the conduct of research and requires such research to be first reviewed by the appropriate institutional review board. The rules shall include the requirement that all researchers sign an oath of confidentiality [California Welfare and Institutions Code § 5328 (e) (Deering 1992)].

California Civil Code § 56.10(c)(7) allows healthcare providers to disclose information to public agencies, clinical investigators, healthcare research organizations, and accredited public or private nonprofit educational or healthcare institutions for bona fide research purposes. However, the recipient may not further disclose the information in any way that would permit identification of the patient.

Research records—in a personal identification form, developed or acquired by any person in the course of conducting research or a research study relating to AIDS—are confidential and the researcher shall not disclose them. Such records are not subject to discovery or production except as provided by law (California Health & Safety Code § 199.30).

Colorado

Colorado Revised Statutes § 27-10-120 notes that records for care and treatment of the mentally ill may be released if the Department of Institutions has promulgated rules for the conduct of research. Such rules shall include the requirement that all researchers sign an oath of confidentiality. All identifying information concerning individual patients—including names, addresses, telephone numbers, and social security numbers—shall not be disclosed for research purposes.

Similarly, records of drug abusers may be made available for research, but the researcher may not publish the results in a way that discloses patients' names or other identifying information (*Id.* § 25-1-1108).

Connecticut

Section 19a-25 makes records procured by the Department of Health Services or by staff committees of facilities accredited by the Department of Health Services in connection with studies of morbidity and mortality confidential and restricts their use to medical or scientific research. No disclosure is authorized except as may be necessary for the purpose of furthering the research project to which it relates.

Section 52-146g provides that a person engaged in research may have access to psychiatric communications and records that identify patients where needed for such research, if such person's research plan is first submitted to and approved by the director of the mental health facility or his or her designee. The communications and records shall not be removed from the mental health facility that prepared them. Coded data or data that does not identify the patient may be removed from a mental health facility, provided the key to the code remains on the premises. The facility and the researcher are responsible for the preservation of the anonymity of the patients.

Delaware

Providers may make information from alcoholism patients' records available for purposes of research into the causes and treatment of alcoholism, but researchers shall not publish such information in a way that discloses patients' names or other identifying information (16 Delaware Code § 2214).

District of Columbia

District of Columbia Code Annotated § 32-255 provides that medical records without names for patients at D.C. General Hospital may be made available to federal, state, and local agencies authorized to conduct utilization review or research with prior consent from the D.C. General Hospital Commission.

Florida

Florida Statutes chapter 381.004(8) allows disclosure of HIV test results to authorized medical or epidemiological researchers, who may not further disclose any identifying characteristics or information.

Information from mental health clinical records may be used for statistical and research purposes if the information is abstracted in such a way as to protect the identity of the patients (Florida Statutes § 394.459).

Georgia

Under Georgia Code § 31-7-6, any hospital, healthcare facility, medical or skilled nursing home, or other organization rendering patient care may provide information, interviews, reports, statements, memoranda, or other data relating to the condition and treatment of any person to research groups approved by the medical staff of the institution involved; governmental health agencies, medical associations and societies; or any in-hospital medical staff committee. Such information may be used in the course of any study for the purpose of reducing rates of morbidity or mortality. No liability of any kind or character for damages or other relief shall arise or be enforced against any person or organization for having provided such information or material, or for having released or published the findings and conclusions of such groups to advance medical research or medical education or to achieve the most effective use of health staffing and facilities, or for having released or published generally a summary of such studies.

The research groups approved by the medical staff of the institution involved—governmental health agencies, medical associations and societies, or any in-hospital medical staff committee—shall use or publish material described in subsection (a) of this code section only for the purposes of advancing medical research or medical education, or to achieve the most effective use of health staffing and facilities, in the interest of reducing rates of morbidity or mortality, except that a summary of such studies may be released by any such group for general publication.

In all events the identity of any person whose condition or treatment has been studied pursuant to this code section shall be confidential and shall not be revealed under any circumstances (*Id.*).

Hawaii

Hawaii's only reference to confidentiality of research data is in Hawaii Revised Statute § 321-43, which provides that mortality and morbidity data of the Department of Health regarding cancer is confidential, except that researchers may use the names of patients to request additional information for research studies when such studies have been approved by the Cancer Commission of the Hawaii Medical Association.

Idaho

Idaho Code § 39-1392b provides that all records are confidential if they relate to research, discipline, or medical study of any in-hospital medical staff committees or medical society. Section 39-1392d adds that all records used in a research discipline or medical study project are the property of the hospital or medical society that obtains or compiles them. In addition, *Id.* § 39-308 provides for an exception to the general rule of confidentiality of records of alcoholics, or of intoxicated or addicted persons receiving treatment. The director may make available information from such records for the purposes of research into the causes and treatment of alcoholism or drug addiction [*Id.* § 39-308 (1)]. However, information from such research shall not be published in a way that discloses patient's names or other identifying information [*Id.* § 39-308(2)].

Illinois

Illinois provides for confidentiality of research information in its peer review statutes, 735 Illinois Compiled Statutes S/8-2101. *See* Chapter 6.

Indiana

See the discussion in Chapter 4 of this book concerning research in communicable disease cases. In addition, Indiana Code § 16-4-2-3 specifies that information and reports received by the state health commissioner are confidential and may be used only for research and medical education. However, such information or reports may not disclose the name or identity of any patient whose records were included in the information so furnished. Section 16-4-2-4 authorizes the state health commissioner to release a summary of a study for the purpose of advancing medical research or medical education but, again, the identity of any person whose condition or treatment was studied is confidential and privileged. The summary may not reveal the patient's identity.

Section 16-4-9-5 contains detailed requirements for the confidentiality of information concerning individual cancer patients and the conditions under which researchers may have access to it, including confidentiality safeguards, as does § 16-4-10-9 with regard to the birth problems registry and § 16-4-11-9 with regard to the traumatic injury registry.

Iowa

Iowa's general statute regarding disclosure for medical research is Iowa Code § 135.40, which provides that any person, hospital, sanatorium, nursing or rest home, or other organization may provide information, interviews, reports, statements, memoranda, or other data relating to the condition and treatment of any person to the Department of Public Health, the Iowa Medical Society or any of its allied medical societies, the Iowa Osteopathic Medical Society, or any in-hospital staff committee to be used in the course of any study for the purpose of reducing morbidity or mortality. The State Department of Health, the Iowa Medical Society or any of its allied medical societies, the Iowa Society of Osteopathic Physicians and Surgeons, or any in-hospital staff committee may use or publish material from any morbidity or mortality studies only to advance medical research or education, except that a summary of such studies may be published. In all events, the identity of any patient will be confidential. Violation of such confidentiality is a misdemeanor (*Id.* § 135.41).

Although § 125.37 makes records of chemical substance abuse confidential, it does however, permit disclosure for purposes of research into the causes and treatment of substance abuse. Such information shall not be published in a way that discloses patients' names or other identifying information.

Section 229.25 specifies that one of the exceptions to the requirement that medical records of mentally ill persons remain confidential is that they may be released by the chief medical officer when requested for the purpose of research into the causes, incidence, nature, and treatment of mental illness. The chief medical officer may release mental health patient records for research purposes so long as he or she does not disclose patient's names or identities (*Id.* § 229.25).

Kansas

Kansas Statutes Annotated § 65-5525(a)(2)(C) provides a specific authorization for disclosure of patients' records for purposes of research into the causes and treatment of drug abuse. Researchers may not publish such information in any way that may disclose a patient's identity.

Similarly, § 65-177 provides for the secretary of health and environment to receive otherwise confidential data in connection with medical research studies conducted for the purpose of reducing morbidity or mortality from maternal, perinatal, and anesthetic causes.

Kentucky

Kentucky has no specific requirements governing access to medical records for research purposes.

Louisiana

Louisiana Revised Statutes 40:3.1 states that all records of interviews, questionnaires, reports, statements, notes, and memoranda, hereafter referred to as "confidential data," procured by and prepared by employees or agents of the Office of Public Health or by any other person, agency, or organization acting jointly with that office, including public or private colleges and universities, in connection with special morbidity and mortality studies and research investigations to determine any cause or condition of health are confidential and shall be used solely for statistical, scientific, and medical research purposes relating to the cause or condition, except as otherwise provided by law.

Any HIV/AIDS testing must for research purposes be performed in such a manner that the identity of the test subject remains anonymous, and the results may not be retrieved by any researcher unless specifically authorized.

Maine

Maine Revised Statutes Title 5, § 19203-D(3) permits access to medical records concerning HIV infection for utilization review and scientific research, provided the individual patient is not identified.

Maryland

Maryland Health-General Code Annotated § 4-102 specifies that state confidential research records may only be used for the research and study for which they were assembled or obtained and may not be disclosed to any person not engaged in the research. However, statistics, information, or other material that summarizes or refers to confidential records in the aggregate without disclosing the identity of any individual may be published.

Massachusetts

Massachusetts General Laws chapter 111, § 24A specifies that all information procured in connection with scientific studies authorized by the commissioner of the Department of Public Health is confidential and shall be used solely for the purposes of medical or scientific research.

Michigan

Michigan Compiled Laws § 333.6113 provides for disclosure of a patient record without the patient's consent to, among others, qualified personnel for the purpose of conducting scientific statistical research, financial audits, or program evaluation, but the personnel shall not directly or indirectly identify an individual.

Section 333.2361 mandates that information of an organization that has been designated as a medical research project by the State Department of Public Health is confidential. Further, data concerning medical research projects is inadmissible in evidence and may not be disclosed except as is necessary for furthering the research (*Id.* § 333.2632).

Minnesota

Minnesota Statutes § 144.053(1) provides that data of the state commissioner of health or of the commissioner and other persons, agencies, and organizations, held jointly, for the purpose of reducing morbidity or mortality is confidential and shall be used solely for the purposes of medical or scientific research. No person participating in the research shall disclose the information except in strict conformity with the research project. Violation of the nondisclosure requirements is a misdemeanor.

Section 254A.09 provides for confidentiality for individuals who are the subject of alcohol or drug abuse research by the state authority.

Mississippi

Mississippi has no specific requirements for disclosure of medical information for research.

Missouri

Revised Statutes of Missouri § 191.656(4) requires that the identity of any subject of HIV testing participating in a research project approved by an institutional review board shall not be reported to the Department of Health by the physician conducting the research project. Under § 192.067, the Department of Health may receive information from patients' medical records for the purpose of conducting epidemiological studies to be used in promoting and safeguarding health but shall maintain the confidentiality of such information.

Montana

Montana Code Annotated § 50-16-529(6) notes that a healthcare provider may disclose healthcare information without the patient's authorization to the extent that the recipient needs to know the information if the disclosure is, among others, for use in a research project that an institutional review board has determined:

- Is of sufficient importance to outweigh the intrusion into the privacy of the patient that would result from disclosure.

- Is impracticable without the use or disclosure of the healthcare information in individually identifiable form.

- Contains reasonable safeguards to protect the information from improper disclosure.

- Contains reasonable safeguards to protect against directly or indirectly identifying any patient in any report of the research project.

- Contains procedures to remove or destroy at the earliest opportunity, consistent with the purposes of the project, information that would enable the patient to be identified, unless an institutional review board authorizes retention of identifying information for purposes of another research project.

Section 50-16-204 adds that in-hospital medical staff committees shall use or publish information from records only for, among other reasons, research and statistical purposes. The name or identity of patients whose records have been studied will not be disclosed.

Section 53-21-166 provides that an exception to the general rule of confidentiality of medical records of the mentally ill is for research, if the Department of Corrections and Human Services has promulgated rules for the conduct of research that include the requirement that all researchers sign an oath of confidentiality.

Section 50-16-102(1) permits use of information on infant morbidity and mortality for advancing medical research or medical education in the interest of reducing infant morbidity or mortality. Such data are privileged but may be given to the Department of Health and Environmental Sciences, the Montana Medical Association, an allied society of the association, a committee of a nationally organized medical society or research group, or an in-hospital staff committee.

Nebraska

Revised Statutes of Nebraska § 71-3402 provides that the Department of Health, the Nebraska State Medical Association, or any of its allied medical societies or any in-hospital staff committee shall only use or publish patient material for the purpose of medical research or education for reducing morbidity and mortality only for those purposes, except that a summary may be released for general publication. In all events, the identity of any person whose condition or treatment has been studied shall be confidential and shall not be revealed under any circumstances.

Nevada

Nevada Revised Statutes Annotated § 457.260(1) allows the health division to make appropriate use of material related to cancer reporting to advance research and education concerning cancer and to improve treatment of the disease.

New Hampshire

New Hampshire Revised Statutes Annotated §§ 318-B:12-a and 172:8-a provides that if the patient makes a written consent, records of drug abuse treatment and records of alcohol and drug abuse treatment may be used for research.

Section 141C:10 specifies conditions under which communicable disease information may be disclosed to researchers. That section requires researchers to demonstrate a need that is essential to health-related research, and any release of information shall be conditioned upon personal identities of patients remaining confidential. Section 141-B:9 contains virtually identical language concerning disclosure of cancer information for research.

New Jersey

Research data provided to the State Department of Health is confidential (New Jersey Statutes § 26:1A-37.2).

New Mexico

Section 14-6-1(c) of New Mexico Statutes Annotated notes that statistical studies and research reports based upon confidential information may be published or released to the public as long as they do not identify individual patients either directly or indirectly or in any way violate the privileged and confidential nature of the relationship and communications between practitioner and patient.

The *New Mexico Hospital Association Handbook* adds that in determining what restrictions should be placed on staff access to medical records for reasons not required by medical care, the hospital must balance the patients' privacy interests against medical staff interest in medical research or the learning value of a particular case. It further adds that without written patient consent, records related to drug and alcohol treatment may be disclosed only to qualified personnel for the purpose of conducting scientific research, management audits, financial audits, or program evaluation, but such personnel may not identify, directly or indirectly, any individual patient in any report of such research or report (Healthcare Financial Management Association, *New Mexico Hospital Association Legal Handbook*, chapter V, § C, ¶ 1-3, at V-6 through V-8).

New Mexico Statutes Annotated §§ 24-2B-1 to 24-2B-8, the Human Immunodeficiency Virus Test Act, permits disclosure of otherwise-confidential test results and the identity of any person tested to authorized medical or epidemiological researchers who may not further disclose any identifying characteristics or information [*Id.* § 24-2B-6(G)].

New York

New York Mental Hygiene Law § 33.13(b) and (c) permit disclosure of confidential mental hygiene client records to qualified researchers upon the approval of an institutional review board or other committee specially constituted for the approval of research projects at the facility, provided that the researcher shall in no event disclose information tending to identify a patient or client.

HIV-related information may be disclosed to health facility staff committees or accreditation or oversight review organizations authorized to access medical records, provided that such committees or organizations may only disclose confidential HIV-related information:

- Back to the facility or provider of a health or social service.
- To carry out the monitoring, evaluation, or service review for which it was obtained.
- To a federal, state, or local government agency for the purpose of monitoring health or social services (*Id.* § 2782).

North Carolina

Confidential communicable disease information, whether publicly or privately maintained, that identifies a person who has AIDS virus infection or who has or may have a reportable disease or condition may be disclosed for bona fide research purposes. Or a provider may release specific medical or epidemiological information for statistical purposes in such a way that no person can be identified (General Statutes of North Carolina § 130A-143).

Section 130A-212 provides that, although the clinical records or reports of cancer patients are confidential, the Commission for Health Services shall provide by rule for their use for medical research.

North Dakota

North Dakota Centennial Code § 23-07.5-05 specifies that a provider of blood may disclose HIV test results to a person who conducts research if the researcher:

- Is affiliated with the test subject's healthcare provider.

- Has obtained permission to perform the research from an institutional review board.

- Provides written assurance to the person disclosing the test results that the information requested is only for the purpose for which it is provided to the research, the information will not be released to a person unconnected with the study, and the final research product will not reveal information that may identify the test subject unless the researcher has first received informed consent for disclosure from the test subject.

Ohio

Ohio Revised Code § 3701.261 permits disclosure of information with respect to a case of malignant disease furnished to a cancer registry for statistical, scientific, and medical research for the purpose of reducing morbidity or mortality. Under § 3793.13, patient records from drug treatment programs may be disclosed without patients' consent to qualified personnel for the purpose of conducting scientific research, management, financial audits, or program evaluation, but these personnel may not identify, directly or indirectly, any individual patient in any report of the research, audit, or evaluation and may not otherwise disclose a patient's identity in any manner.

Oklahoma

Oklahoma Statutes Annotated Title 63, § 1-1709 specifies that any authorized person, hospital, sanatorium, nursing home, rest home, or other organization may provide information relating to the condition and treatment of any person to the State Board of Health; the Oklahoma State Medical Association, or any committee or allied society thereof; the American Medical Association, other national organization approved by the State Board of Health, or any committee or allied medical society thereof; or any in-hospital staff committee for use in studies for the purpose of reducing morbidity or mortality. Recipients shall use or publish such information or material only for the purpose of advancing medical research or education in the interest of reducing morbidity or mortality, except that a summary of such studies may be released for general publication.

In all events, the identity of any person whose condition or treatment has been studied shall be confidential and not revealed under any circumstances. Any information furnished shall not contain the name of the person upon whom information is furnished and shall not violate the confidential relationship of patient and doctor. All such information and the findings and conclusions of such studies are privileged and not admissible in evidence (*Id.*).

Oregon

Under Oregon Revised Statutes § 179.505(4)(b), a public healthcare provider may release, without patient consent, written medical records such as case histories, clinical records, X-rays, progress reports, treatment charts, and other similar patient records maintained by the provider to persons engaged in scientific research, at the discretion of the responsible officer.

The provider shall not disclose patient identities except when essential to the research. When a patient's identity is disclosed, the provider shall include in the patient's permanent record a written statement detailing the reasons for the disclosure, what was disclosed, and recipients of the information [*Id.* § 179.505(5)].

Pennsylvania

Pennsylvania has no specific requirements concerning disclosure of medical record information for research.

Rhode Island

The Confidentiality of Health Care Information Act provides for disclosure of medical records to qualified researchers, auditors, and so on, provided they do not identify any individual patient in any report, audit, or evaluation or otherwise disclose patient identities [Rhode Island General Laws § 5-37.3-4(b)(3)].

The director of an alcoholism treatment facility may make information from alcoholism patients' records available for research into the causes and treatment of alcoholism, but researchers may not publish information in a way that discloses patients' names or other identifying information.

South Carolina

South Carolina Code Annotated § 44-1-110 permits the Department of Health and Environmental Control to investigate the causes, character, and means of preventing the epidemic and endemic diseases from which patients within the state may suffer. Thus, the department has, upon request, full access to the medical records, tumor registries, and other special disease records systems maintained by physicians, hospitals, and other health facilities as necessary to carry out its investigation of these diseases. The department must keep patient-identifying information confidential.

Section 44-52-190(3), which establishes confidentiality of records that identify drug and alcohol abuse patients, permits disclosure for research conducted or authorized by the State Department of Mental Health or the South Carolina Commission on Alcohol and Drug Abuse. Section 44-52-170(f) permits disclosure in the same circumstances of records of such patients' commitment.

Section 44-29-135, which mandates confidentiality of records regarding sexually transmitted diseases, permits disclosure of medical or epidemiological information for statistical purposes in a manner that does not reveal the identity of any person.

Concerning the statewide Alzheimer's disease and related disorders registry, the School of Public Health and all persons to whom data is released shall keep all patient information confidential. No publication of information, biomedical research, or medical data may identify the patients (*Id.* § 44-36-30).

South Dakota

Section 34-14-1 makes information procured in the course of a medical study strictly confidential and specifies that it may only be used for medical research. Disclosure of information from a medical study constitutes a misdemeanor (*Id.* § 34-14-3).

Tennessee

Under Tennessee Code Annotated § 68-10-113(1), records or information concerning sexually transmitted disease held by health departments are confidential but may be released for statistical purposes in such a form that no individual person can be identified.

Section 68-3-504 specifies that reports of fetal deaths are to be used only for medical, health, and research purposes.

Texas

Section 161.022 provides for confidentiality of information used in medical research and education. Texas Revised Civil Statute article 4495b, § 5.08(n)(3) lists as one of the exceptions to the physician-patient privilege, disclosure to qualified personnel for research, but research personnel may not identify, directly or indirectly, a patient in any report of the research or otherwise disclose identity in any manner.

Under Texas Health and Safety Code Annotated § 161.021(a), a person, including a hospital, nursing home, medical society, or other organization, may provide information to various organizations and practitioners relating to the condition and treatment of any person for studies to reduce morbidity or mortality or to identify persons who may need immunization. The recipients may only use such data to advance medical research or medical education in the interest of reducing morbidity or mortality, except that they may release a summary of the studies for general publication. However, the identity of a person whose condition or treatment has been studied is confidential and may not be revealed except to identify persons who need immunization. The information and any findings or conclusions resulting from that study are privileged [*Id.* § 161.022(b) and (c)].

A person may disclose test results of AIDS, HIV, or other related disorders for statistical summary purposes only without the written consent of the person tested if he or she removes information that could identify the subject [*Id.* § 81.103(e)].

Utah

Utah Code Annotated § 26-25-1 states that any person or health facility may, without incurring liability, provide information, interviews, reports, statements, memoranda, or other data relating to the condition and treatment of any person to the Department of Health, to the Division of Mental Health within the Department of Social Services, to research organizations, to peer review committees, to professional review organizations, to professional societies and associations, or to any health facility's in-house staff committee for use in any study with the purpose of reducing morbidity or mortality or for the evaluation and improvement of hospital and health care. Such data is confidential and privileged. Section 26-25-2 provides that the Department of Health; the Division of Mental Health of the Department of Human Services; scientific and healthcare research organizations affiliated with institutions of higher education; the Utah State Medical Association or any of its allied medical societies, peer review committees, professional review organizations, professional societies and associations;

or any health facility's in-house staff committee may only use or publish data received or gathered under § 26-25-1 for the purpose of advancing medical research or medical education in the interest of reducing morbidity or mortality, except that a summary of studies may be released for general publication.

Section 26-25a-101(2)(b), (c), and (e) through (i) provide that specific medical or epidemiological information regarding communicable or reportable diseases may be released to authorized personnel within the Department of Health, local health departments, official health agencies in other states, the U.S. Public Health Service, or the Centers for Disease Control, when necessary to continue patient services or to undertake public health efforts to interrupt the transmission of disease, presumably including research.

Section 62A-4-513(1)(g) provides that otherwise-confidential child abuse reports and information may be disclosed to a person engaged in bona fide research, when approved by the director of the division, if the information does not contain names and addresses.

Vermont

Vermont's Bill of Rights for Hospital Patients, contained in Vermont Statutes Annotated Title 18, § 1852(7), notes that in regards to a patient's right to privacy, medical personnel or individuals under the supervision of medical personnel who are researching the effectiveness of that medical treatment shall have access to the patient's medical records without the patient's consent.

Virginia

Virginia Code Annotated §§ 42.48.020 and 42.48.040 provide for the confidentiality of records used for research purposes. Section 32.1-36.1(A)(6), which provides for confidentiality of tests for HIV, specifies that such test results may be released to medical or epidemiological researchers for use as statistical data only.

Section 32.1-40 permits the commissioner of health or his or her designee to examine and review any medical records in the course of investigation, research, or studies of diseases or deaths of public health importance. Section 32.1-41 requires the commissioner or his or her designee to preserve the anonymity of each patient and practitioner of the healing arts whose records are examined pursuant to § 32.1-41, except that the commissioner, in his or her sole discretion, may divulge the identity of such patients and practitioners if pertinent to an investigation, research, or study. Any person to whom such identities are divulged shall preserve their anonymity.

Section 32.1-74.4 makes confidential the information released to the commissioner of health concerning Alzheimer's disease and related disorders. No publication of information, biomedical research, or medical data shall identify the patients.

Washington

Revised Code of Washington § 42.48.020(1) provides that a state agency may authorize, provide access to, or provide copies of an individually identifiable personal record for research purposes if informed written consent for the disclosure has been given to the appropriate department secretary, the president of the institution, or his or her designee, by the person to whom the record pertains, or, in the case of minors and legally incompetent adults, the person's legally authorized representative. This statute also provides detailed guidelines for such disclosure without patient consent [*Id.* § 42.48.020(2)]. In addition, § 42.48.040 provides for confidentiality of research records and specifies the conditions under which individually identifiable records may be disclosed. Unauthorized disclosure is a misdemeanor (*Id.* § 42.48.050).

Section 70.96A.150(2) and (3) permits the secretary of the Department of Social and Health Services to receive information from alcoholic and intoxicated patients' records for purposes of research into the causes and treatment of alcoholism and other drug addiction, verification of eligibility and appropriateness of reimbursement, and the evaluation of alcoholism and other drug treatment programs. Such information shall not be published in a way that discloses patients' names or identities. Section 71.05.630 permits disclosure of mental illness patient records for research.

West Virginia

West Virginia Code § 16-3C-2(e)(2) permits disclosure of the performance of an HIV-related test for the purpose of research if the testing is performed in a manner by which the identity of the test subject is not known and may not be retrieved by the researcher.

Wisconsin

Wisconsin Statutes § 146.82(2)(b), governing confidentiality of healthcare records, permits access without informed consent for purposes of research if the researcher is affiliated with the healthcare provider and provides written assurances to the custodian of the patient healthcare records that the information will be used only for the purposes for which it is provided to the researcher, the information will not be released to a person unconnected with the study, and the final product of the research will not reveal information that may serve to identify the patient whose records are being released without the informed consent of the patient. The private-pay patient may deny such access by annually submitting to the healthcare provider a signed, written request on a form provided by the Department of Health and Social Services.

Wisconsin Administrative Code § HSS 92.04(3) (June 1986), relating to confidentiality of treatment records of persons treated for mental illness, developmental disabilities, and alcohol or drug abuse, permits access to medical records without patient consent for authorized research.

Section 146.025(4), relating to confidentiality of AIDS testing information, permits use of confidential data for research if the researcher is affiliated with a healthcare provider, has obtained permission to perform the research from an institutional review board, and provides written assurance to the person disclosing the tests results that use of the information is limited to the purpose provided by the researcher, the information will not be released to a person unconnected with the study, and the final research product will not reveal information that may identify the subject unless the researcher has first received informed consent for disclosure from the subject.

Wyoming

Under Wyoming Statutes § 35-2-609(a)(vii), a hospital may disclose healthcare information about a patient without the patient's authorization to the extent that the recipient needs to know the information for use in a research project that an institutional review board has determined:

- Is of sufficient importance to outweigh the intrusion into the privacy of the patient that would result from the disclosure.

- Is impracticable without the use or disclosure of healthcare information in individual identifiable form.

- Contains reasonable safeguards to protect against identifying, directly or indirectly, any patient in any report of the research project.

- Contains procedures to remove or destroy at the earliest possible opportunity, consistent with the purposes of the project, information that would enable the patient to be identified, unless an institutional review board authorizes retention of identifying information for purposes of another research project.

In addition, subject to bylaws and control by the hospital governing body, the medical staff committees of any hospital shall have access to the records, data, and other information relating to the condition and treatment of patients in that hospital for the purpose of evaluating, studying, and reporting on matters relating to the care and treatment of patients and for research; reducing mortality; and prevention and treatment of diseases, illnesses and injuries [*Id.* § 35-2-609(c)].

Conclusion

Just because a researcher has used patient information in a research project does not destroy the confidential nature of that information. Although the researcher may use such information, he or she should obtain informed consent to use it, if possible, even if a statute provides for such disclosure, and he or she must protect the identities of the subjects of the research.

6

Confidentiality of Peer Review Information

Introduction

Peer review information is perhaps unique in that patients *and* practitioners have interests both in keeping such information confidential and in disclosure. Patients want information about their cases treated confidentially yet may want access to the minutes or records of peer review meetings discussing their case because, given the type of open discussion that should occur during a peer review meeting, the records of the review could be helpful to a plaintiff suing either the physician under review or the health-care facility. Likewise, a physician who was denied staff privileges or otherwise sanctioned by a credentials committee could use these materials to contest the action. A fear that what they say might be used in malpractice litigation could deter peer review participants from being totally candid.

One court noted that "confidentiality is essential to effective functioning of these staff meetings, and these staff meetings are essential to the continued improvement in the care and treatment of patients."[1]

Competing against this interest, however, is the patient's interest in learning whether he or she was the victim of medical incompetence. As another court said, "This confidentiality exacts a social cost because it impairs a malpractice plaintiff's access to evidence. Such unavailability of recorded evidence of malpractice might seriously jeopardize or even prevent the plaintiff's recovery."[2]

In the balancing test, however, between the general public's need for the benefits of peer review and the individual patient's interest, the legislatures generally uphold the greater public policy interest of ensuring good health care to the whole of society over the individual patient's concerns. Thus, most legislatures have enacted statutes providing for confidentiality of peer review information. Federal laws do not discuss confidentiality of peer review information as comprehensively as do the states.

Federal Laws

The Health Care Quality Improvement Act of 1986 requires reporting of incompetent physicians. The act provides that the reported information is confidential but does not provide any confidentiality protection for peer review activities.[3]

The statute creating peer review organizations (PROs) under the Utilization and Quality Control Peer Review Organization Program (see Chapter 2) provides for limited confidentiality for PRO information. PROs may disclose information showing the mortality rate, by hospital, for various types of surgery and the number of patients who develop postoperative infections, the average length-of-stay, and the cost of various procedures. They may disclose hospital identities but not the names of individual physicians. PROs may also disclose their opinion concerning the quality of care at particular hospitals.[4]

State Laws

Because of the failure of the Health Care Quality Improvement Act to provide for the confidentiality of review activities, one must look primarily at state statutes to determine the existence and extent of any protection from disclosure of peer review information. As with immunity issues, state statutes vary widely in scope of the privilege against disclosure of peer review information. Some states provide absolute confidentiality with respect to peer review materials. Typically, these states use a statute that provides that records of peer review committees are not subject to discovery or introduction into evidence in any civil action against a provider of professional health services arising out of matters that are the subject of the committee's evaluation and review. Other state statutes add that such materials are not subject to subpoena. Still other states, however, provide only limited protection.

For example, Nebraska provides that a plaintiff may not discover peer review materials unless he or she waives the privilege against disclosure and a court, after a hearing and for good cause arising from extraordinary circumstances, orders the disclosure.[5]

What are "peer review materials" for the purpose of confidentiality provisions? Some state statutes are vague in defining the scope of these materials, which leaves it to the courts to determine. If a court reads the term narrowly, a plaintiff may be able to discover some peer review information. Other state confidentiality statutes are quite explicit. Idaho, for example, protects "all written records of interviews, all reports, statements, minutes, memoranda, charts, and the contents thereof, and all physical materials relating to research, discipline, or medical study of any in-hospital medical staff committees or medical society."[6]

Some states also provide an exception to the general rule against discovery of peer review materials that allows a physician who is challenging his or her curtailment, suspension, termination, or denial of staff privileges to obtain access to peer review materials.[7]

However, even if the information is not discoverable, that doesn't always answer the question of whether a participant in a peer review activity may testify about peer review proceedings. Some states permit the peer reviewer to testify voluntarily about peer review proceedings but prohibit required testimony. Others permit physicians involved in peer review to testify about their professional opinions but not about specific details of the peer review proceedings.[8]

Alabama

Information provided to any peer review committee and any findings, conclusions, or recommendations of such a committee are privileged and confidential (*Id.* § 6-5-333).

Alaska

Alaska Statutes provide that all data and information acquired by a peer review organization in the exercise of its duties is confidential and may not be disclosed except to the extent necessary to carry out its functions. Nor is such information subject to subpoena. However, healthcare providers aggrieved by a peer review committee may have access to such information.[9]

Arizona

Arizona Revised Statutes § 36-445.01 specifies confidentiality of peer review information and conditions of disclosure. All proceedings, records, and materials prepared in connection with peer reviews, including all peer reviews of individual healthcare providers practicing in and applying to practice in hospitals or outpatient surgical centers and the records of such reviews, shall be confidential and shall not be subject to discovery except in proceedings before the Board of Medical Examiners, or the Board of Osteopathic Examiners, or in actions by an individual healthcare provider against a hospital or center or its medical staff arising from discipline of such individual healthcare provider or refusal, termination, suspension, or limitation of his or her privileges. No member of a committee established under the provisions of § 36-445 (to review the professional practices within the hospital or center for the purposes of reducing morbidity and mortality and for the improvement of the care of patients) or officer or other member of a hospital's or center's medical, administrative, or nursing staff engaged in assisting the hospital or center to carry out functions in accordance with that section or any person furnishing information to a committee performing peer review may be subpoenaed to testify in any judicial or quasi-judicial proceeding if such subpoena is based solely on such activities.

Arkansas

Arkansas Code § 20-9-503 makes confidential the proceeding and records of peer review committees.

California

California Evidence Code § 1157 states that neither the proceedings nor the records of any of the following are subject to discovery:

- Organized committees of medical, medical-dental, podiatric, registered dietitian, psychological, or veterinary staffs in hospitals.

- Peer review bodies, having the responsibility of evaluation and improvement of the quality of care rendered in the hospital.

- For those peer review bodies, or medical or dental review or dental hygienist review or chiropractic review or podiatric review or registered dietitian review or veterinary review committees of local medical, dental, dental hygienist, podiatric, dietetic, veterinary, or chiropractic societies, or psychological review committees of state or local psychological associations or societies having the responsibility of evaluation and improvement of the quality of care, shall be subject to discovery.

Colorado

Any information, data, reports, or records made available to a utilization review committee of a hospital or other healthcare facility, as required by state or federal law, are confidential and shall be used by such committee and the members thereof only in the exercise of the proper functions of the committee. It shall not be a violation of a privileged communication for any physician, dentist, podiatrist, hospital, or other healthcare facility or person to furnish information, data, reports, or records to any such utilization review committee concerning any patient examined or treated by the same or confined in such hospital or facility, which information, data, reports, or records relate to the proper functions of the utilization review committee (Colorado Statutes § 13-21-110).

Connecticut

The proceedings of a medical review committee conducting a peer review shall not be subject to discovery or introduction into evidence in any civil action for or against a healthcare provider arising out of the matters that are subject to evaluation and review by such committee, and no person who was in attendance at a meeting of such committee shall be permitted or required to testify in any such civil action about the content of such proceedings, provided the provisions of this subsection shall not preclude:

- In any civil action, the use of any writing that was recorded independently of such proceedings.

- In any civil action, the testimony of any person concerning the facts that formed the basis for the institution of such proceedings of which he or she had personal knowledge acquired independently of such proceedings.

- In any healthcare provider proceedings concerning the termination or restriction of staff privileges, other than peer review, the use of data discussed or developed during peer review proceedings.

- In any civil action, disclosure of the fact that staff privileges were terminated or restricted, including the specific restrictions imposed, if any (Connecticut General Statutes § 19a-17b).

Delaware

The records and proceedings of the Board of Medical Practice, the Medical Society of Delaware, their members, or the members of any committees appointed thereby or the members of any committee appointed by a certified health maintenance organization, and members of hospital and osteopathic medical society committees, or of a professional standards review organization established under federal law (or other peer review committee or organization), whose function is the review of medical records, medical care, and physicians' work, with a view to the quality of care and utilization of hospital or nursing home facilities, home visits, and office visits, shall be confidential and shall be used by such committees or organizations and the members thereof only in the exercise of the proper functions of the committee or organization and shall not be public records and shall not be available for court subpoena or subject to discovery (16 Delaware Code § 1768).

District of Columbia

Any publication by any medical utilization review committee, peer review committee, medical staff committee, or tissue review committee shall keep confidential the identity of any patient whose condition, care or treatment was a part thereof (District of Columbia Code § 32-504).

Absent a showing of extraordinary necessity, the minutes, analyses, preliminary and final findings, and reports of a medical utilization review committee, peer review committee, medical staff committee, or tissue review committee shall not be subject to discovery or admissible into evidence in any civil or administrative proceeding. This qualified privilege does not extend to primary health records or to any oral or written statements submitted to or presented before a medical utilization review committee, peer review committee, medical staff committee, or tissue review committee.

This statute does not affect the right of any individual employed by or formerly employed by a hospital or extended care facility operating within the District of Columbia; a professional medical society or psychological association operating within the district; a medical school engaged in research within the district; a department, agency, or instrumentality of the federal government operating within the district; a department or agency of the district government to admit into evidence or subject to discovery the minutes and reports of a medical utilization review committee, peer review committee, medical staff committee, or tissue review committee for the limited purpose of adjudicating the appropriateness of an adverse action affecting the employment, work, or association or the termination of employment, work, or association of such person (*Id.* § 32-505).

Florida

The investigations, proceedings, and records of a peer review committee are not subject to discovery or introduction into evidence in any civil or administrative action against a provider of professional health services arising out of the matters that are the subject of evaluation and review by such committee. However, information, documents, or records otherwise available from original sources are not to be construed as immune from discovery or use in any such civil action merely because they were presented during proceedings of such committee (Florida Statutes § 766.101).

Georgia

Code of Georgia § 31-7-133 provides for confidentiality of review organizations' records. The proceedings and records of a review organization shall be held in confidence and shall not be subject to discovery or introduction into evidence in any civil action arising out of or otherwise directly related to the matters that are the subject of evaluation and review by such organization. However, information, documents, or records otherwise available from original sources are not to be construed as immune from discovery or use in any such civil action merely because they were presented during proceedings of such an organization.

Under § 31-7-143, the proceedings and records of medical review committees shall not be subject to discovery or introduction into evidence in any civil action against a provider of professional health services arising out of the matters that are the subject of evaluation and review by such committee. However, information, documents, or records otherwise available from original sources shall not be construed as immune from discovery or use in any such civil action merely because they were presented during proceedings of such committee.

Hawaii

Neither the proceedings nor the records of peer review committees, hospital committees, or clinic quality assurance committees are subject to discovery. For the purposes of this statute, "records of hospital committees or clinic quality assurance committees" are limited to recordings, transcripts, minutes, summaries, and reports of committee meetings and conclusions contained therein. Protected information does not include incident reports, occurrence reports, or similar reports that state facts concerning a specific situation, or records made in the regular course of business by a hospital or other healthcare provider. Original sources of information, documents, or records shall not be immune from discovery or use in any civil proceeding merely because they were presented to, or prepared at the direction of, such committees (Hawaii Statutes § 624-25.5).

Idaho

Idaho Code § 39-1392 states that to encourage research, discipline, and medical study by in-hospital medical staff committees and recognized medical societies for the purposes of reducing morbidity and mortality, enforcing and improving the standards of medical practice in the state of Idaho, certain records of such committees and societies shall be confidential and privileged.

Under § 39-1392b, records of such entities are confidential and privileged. Except as provided in section 39-1392e, all written records of interviews; all reports, statements, minutes, memoranda, charts, and the contents thereof; and all physical materials relating to research, discipline, or medical study of any in-hospital medical staff committees or medical society, for the purposes set forth in § 39-1392, are confidential and privileged, and shall not be directly or indirectly subject to subpoena or discovery proceedings, or be admitted as evidence.

Illinois

All information, interviews, reports, statements, memoranda, or other data of the Illinois Department of Public Health, municipal health departments, the Illinois Department of Mental Health and Developmental Disabilities, the Mental Health and Developmental Disabilities Medical Review Board, Illinois State Medical Society, allied medical societies, health maintenance organizations, medical organizations under contract with health maintenance organizations, physician-owned interinsurance exchanges and their agents, or committees of licensed or accredited hospitals or their medical staffs, including Patient Care Audit Committees, Medical Care Evaluation Committees, Utilization Review Committees, Credential Committees, and Executive Committees (but not the medical records pertaining to the patient) used in the course of internal quality control or of medical study for the purpose of reducing morbidity or mortality, or for improving patient care, shall be privileged and strictly confidential, and shall be used only for medical research; the evaluation and improvement of quality care; or granting, limiting, or revoking staff privileges, except that in any hospital proceeding to decide upon a physician's staff privileges or any judicial review thereof, the claim of confidentiality shall not be invoked to deny such physician access to or use of data upon which such a decision was based (735 Illinois Compiled Statutes 5/8-2101).

Under 735 Illinois Compiled Statutes 5/8-2102, such information, records, reports, statements, notes, memoranda, or other data shall not be admissible as evidence nor discoverable in any action of any kind in any court or before any tribunal, board, agency, or person. The disclosure of any such information or data, whether proper or improper, shall not waive or have any effect upon its confidentiality, nondiscoverability, or nonadmissibility.

Indiana

Indiana Code § 34-4-12.6-2 specifies that all proceedings of a peer review committee shall be confidential. All communications to a peer review committee shall be privileged communications. Neither the personnel of a peer review committee nor any participant in a committee proceeding shall reveal any content of communications to, the records of, or the determination of a peer review committee outside the peer committee.

Communications to, records of, and determinations of a peer review committee may only be disclosed to:

- The peer review committee of a hospital or other health facility.
- The disciplinary authority of the professional organization of which the professional healthcare provider under question is a member.
- The appropriate state board of registration and licensure that the committee considers necessary for recommended disciplinary action and shall otherwise be kept confidential for use only within the scope of the committee's work, unless the professional healthcare provider has filed a prior written waiver of confidentiality with the peer review committee.

Except in cases of required disclosure to the professional healthcare provider under investigation, no records from, determinations of, or communications to a peer review committee shall be:

- Subject to subpoena or discovery.
- Admissible in evidence in any judicial or administrative proceeding without a prior waiver executed by the committee.

Iowa

Peer review records are privileged and confidential; are not subject to discovery, subpoena, or other means of legal compulsion for release to a person other than an affected licensee or a peer review committee; and are not admissible in evidence in a judicial or administrative proceeding other than one involving licensee discipline or a proceeding brought by a licensee who is the subject of a peer review record and whose competence is at issue (Iowa Code § 147.1).

Under § 331.532, the release or publication of a record of the proceedings or of the reports, findings, and conclusions of a review entity shall be for one or more of the following purposes:

- To advance healthcare research or healthcare education.

- To maintain the standards of the healthcare professions.

- To protect the financial integrity of any governmentally funded program.

- To provide evidence relating to the ethics or discipline of a healthcare provider, entity, or practitioner.

- To review the qualifications, competence, and performance of a healthcare professional with respect to the selection and appointment of the healthcare professional to the medical staff of a health facility.

The identity of a person whose condition or treatment has been studied under this act is confidential, and a review entity shall remove the person's name and address from the record before the review entity releases or publishes a record of its proceedings, or its reports, findings, and conclusions. Except as otherwise provided in the preceding paragraph, the record of a proceeding and the reports, findings, and conclusions of a review entity and data collected by or for a review entity under this act are confidential, are not public records, and are not discoverable and shall not be used as evidence in a civil action or administrative proceeding (*Id.* § 331.533).

Kansas

Except as provided by Kansas Statutes Annotated § 60-437 (relating to waiver of a privilege by contract or by previous disclosure) and the exceptions that follow, the reports, statements, memoranda, proceedings, findings, and other records of peer review committees or officers shall be privileged and shall not be subject to discovery, subpoena, or other means of legal compulsion for their release to any person or entity or be admissible in evidence in any judicial or administrative proceeding. Information contained in such records shall not be discoverable or admissible at trial in the form of testimony by an individual who participated in the peer review process. This privilege may be claimed by the legal entity creating the peer review committee or officer, or by the commissioner of insurance for any records or proceedings of the board of governors (Kansas Statutes Annotated § 65-4915).

This privilege shall not apply to proceedings in which a healthcare provider contests the revocation, denial, restriction, or termination of staff privileges or the license, registration, certification, or other authorization to practice of the healthcare provider. Nothing in this statute limits the authority, which may otherwise be provided by law, of the commissioner of insurance, the state board of healing arts, or other healthcare licensing or disciplinary boards of this state to require a peer review committee or officer to report to it any disciplinary action or recommendation of such committee or officer; to transfer to it records of such committee's or officer's proceedings or actions to restrict or revoke the license, registration, certification, or other authorization to practice of a healthcare provider; or to terminate the liability of the fund for all claims against a specific healthcare provider for damages for death or personal injury.

Reports and records so furnished shall not be subject to discovery, subpoena, or other means of legal compulsion for their release to any person or entity and shall not be admissible in evidence in any judicial or administrative proceeding other than a disciplinary proceeding by the state board of healing arts or other healthcare provider licensing or disciplinary boards of this state (*Id.*).

Kentucky

At all times in performing a designated professional review function, the proceedings, records, opinions, conclusions, and recommendations of any committee, board, commission, medical staff, professional standards review organization, or other entity are confidential and privileged and are not subject to discovery, subpoena, or introduction into evidence in any civil action in any court or in any administrative proceeding before any board, body, or committee—whether federal, state, county, or city—except as specifically provided with regard to the board in Kentucky Revised Statutes § 311.605(2) (pertaining to proceedings for violations of licensure rules). This statute does not apply to any proceedings or matters governed exclusively by federal law or federal regulation (Kentucky Revised Statutes § 311.377).

Section 211.463(c) provides that a private agent charged with utilization review may not disclose or publish individual medical records or any other confidential medical information in the performance of utilization review activities except that private review agents may, if otherwise permitted by law, provide patient information to a third party on whose behalf the private review agent is performing utilization review. Section § 211.464(b) requires that private review agents charged with utilization review include in their applications a utilization review plan that includes the policies and procedures that will ensure compliance with all applicable state and federal laws to protect the confidentiality of individual medical records.

Louisiana

Louisiana's medical records confidentiality law provides that the records and proceedings of any public hospital committee, medical organization committee, or extended care facility committee established under state or federal law or regulations or under the bylaws, rules, or regulations of such organization or institution or of any hospital committee, medical organizational committee, or extended care facility committee established by a licensed private hospital are confidential and shall be used by such committee and the members thereof only in the exercise of the proper functions of the committee and shall not be public records and shall not be available for court subpoena. Nothing contained in this statute prevents disclosure of such data to appropriate state or federal regulatory agencies that by statute or regulation are otherwise entitled to access to such data (Louisiana Revised Statutes § 44:7).

Section 3715.3 provides for confidentiality of peer review committee records.

Maine

All proceedings and records of review committees are confidential and are exempt from discovery without a showing of good cause (Maine Revised Statutes Title 32, § 3296).

Maryland

Proceedings, records, and files of medical review committees are confidential and not admissible or discoverable. Except as otherwise provided, the proceedings, records, and files of a medical review committee are not discoverable and are not admissible in evidence in any civil action arising out of matters that are being reviewed and evaluated by the medical review committee (Code of Maryland § 14-501).

The proceedings, records, and files of a medical review committee requested by the Department of Health and Mental Hygiene are confidential and are neither discoverable nor admissible in evidence in any civil action arising out of matters that are being reviewed and evaluated by the medical review committee (*Id.*).

The privilege does not apply to:

- A civil action brought by a party to the proceedings of the medical review committee who claims to be aggrieved by the decision of the medical review committee.

- Any record or document that is considered by the medical review committee and that otherwise would be subject to discovery and introduction into evidence in a civil trial *(Id.)*.

Massachusetts

Under Massachusetts General Laws chapter 111, § 204, except as otherwise provided in the following, the proceedings, reports, and records of a medical peer review committee are confidential and are not subject to subpoena or discovery, or introduced into evidence in any judicial or administrative proceeding, except proceedings held by the boards of registration in medicine, social work, or psychology.

Documents, incident reports or records, otherwise available from original sources are immune from subpoena, discovery, or use in any such judicial or administrative proceeding merely because they were presented to such committee in connection with its proceedings. Nor shall the proceedings, reports, findings, and records of a medical peer review committee be immune from subpoena, discovery, or use as evidence in any proceeding against a member of such committee to establish a cause of action pursuant to chapter 231, § 85N (damages as a result of acts within the scope of one's committee duties); provided, however, that in no event shall the identity of any person furnishing information or opinions to the committee be disclosed without the permission of such person. Nor shall the provisions of this section apply to any investigation or administrative proceeding conducted by the boards of registration in medicine, social work, or psychology *(Id.)*.

Michigan

Under Michigan Compiled Laws § 331.532, the release or publication of a record of the proceedings or of the reports, findings, and conclusions of a review entity shall be for one or more of the following purposes:

- To advance healthcare research or healthcare education.

- To maintain the standards of the healthcare professions.

- To protect the financial integrity of any governmentally funded program.

- To provide evidence relating to the ethics or discipline of a healthcare provider, entity, or practitioner.

- To review the qualifications, competence, and performance of a healthcare professional with respect to the selection and appointment of the healthcare professional to the medical staff of a health facility.

The identity of a person whose condition or treatment has been studied under this act is confidential, and a review entity shall remove the person's name and address from the record before the review entity releases or publishes a record of its proceedings or its reports, findings, and conclusions. Except as otherwise provided, the record of a proceeding and the reports, findings, and conclusions of a review entity and data collected by or for a review entity under this act are confidential, are not public records, are not discoverable, and shall not be used as evidence in a civil action or administrative proceeding (*Id.* § 331.533).

Minnesota

All data and information acquired by a review organization, in the exercise of its duties and functions, shall be held in confidence, shall not be disclosed to anyone except to the extent necessary to carry out one or more of the purposes of the review organization, and shall not be subject to subpoena or discovery. The proceedings and records of a review organization shall not be subject to discovery or introduction into evidence in any civil action against a professional arising out of the matter or matters that are the subject of consideration by the review organization. Information, documents, or records otherwise available from original sources shall not be immune from discovery or use in any civil action merely because they were presented during proceedings of a review organization.

The confidentiality protection and protection from discovery or introduction into evidence also applies to the governing body of the review organization and shall not be waived as a result of referral of a matter from the review organization to the governing body or consideration by the governing body of decisions, recommendations, or documentation of the review organization. These restrictions do not apply to professionals requesting or seeking through discovery, data, information, or records relating to their medical staff privileges, membership, or participation status. However, any data so disclosed in such proceedings shall not be admissible in any other judicial proceeding than those brought by the professional to challenge an action relating to the professional's medical staff privileges or participation status (Minnesota Statutes § 145.64).

Mississippi

Under the Mississippi Code § 41-63-3, data and records provided to a medical or dental association or staff committee shall not divulge the identity of any patient.

Section 41-63-7 notes that the identity of any person whose condition or treatment has been studied by a review committee shall be confidential and shall not be revealed under any circumstances. Any person who reveals the identity of such person in violation of this subsection shall be guilty of a misdemeanor, and upon conviction thereof, shall be subject to confinement in the county jail for a term not to exceed one year and fined a sum not to exceed $500.

Under § 41-83-17, private review agents may not disclose or publish individual medical records or other confidential medical information obtained in the performance of utilization review activities without the patient's authorization or a court order.

Missouri

Except as otherwise provided, the proceedings, findings, deliberations, reports, and minutes of peer review committees concerning the health care provided to any patient are privileged and shall not be subject to discovery, subpoena, or other means of legal compulsion for their release to any person or entity or be admissible into evidence in any judicial or administrative action for failure to provide appropriate care (Missouri Statutes § 537.035).

The provisions limiting discovery and admissibility of the proceedings, findings, records, and minutes of peer review committees do not apply in any judicial or administrative action brought by a peer review committee or the legal entity that formed or within which such committee operates to deny, restrict, or revoke the hospital staff privileges or license to practice of a physician or other healthcare provider. Nor do they apply when a member, employee, or agent of the peer review committee or the legal entity that formed such committee or within which such a committee operates is sued for actions taken by such committee *(Id.)*.

Neither does anything in this statute limit the authority of a healthcare licensing board to obtain information by subpoena or other authorized process from peer review committees or to require disclosure of otherwise-confidential information relating to matters and investigations within the jurisdiction of such healthcare licensing boards *(Id.)*.

Montana

Under Montana Code § 37-2-201, the proceedings and records of professional utilization, peer review, medical ethics review, and professional standards review committees are not subject to discovery or introduction into evidence in any proceeding. However, information otherwise discoverable or admissible from an original source is not immune from discovery or use in any proceeding merely because it was presented during proceedings before the committee, nor is a member of the committee or other person appearing before it to be prevented from testifying about matters within his or her knowledge, but the person cannot be questioned about his or her testimony or other proceedings before the committee or about opinions or other actions of the committee or any member thereof.

This statute also applies to any member, agent, or employee of a non-profit corporation engaged in performing the functions of a peer review, medical ethics review, or professional standards review committee (*Id.*).

Section 50-16-203 makes committee information and proceedings confidential and privileged. All such records, data, and information shall be confidential and privileged to said committee and the members thereof, as though such hospital patients were the patients of the members of such committee. All proceedings and in-hospital records and reports of such medical staff committees shall be confidential and privileged.

Such in-hospital medical staff committees shall use or publish information from such material only for the purpose of evaluating matters of medical care, therapy, and treatment for research and statistical purposes. Neither such in-hospital medical staff committee nor the members, agents, or employees thereof shall disclose the name or identity of any patient whose records have been studied in any report or publication of findings and conclusions of such committee, but such in-hospital medical staff committee, its members, agents, or employees shall protect the identity of any patient whose condition or treatment has been studied and shall not disclose or reveal the name of any such in-hospital patient (*Id.* § 50-16-204).

Nebraska

The proceedings and records of a peer review committee of a state or local association or society composed of licensed health practitioners shall be held in confidence and shall not be subject to discovery or introduction into evidence in any civil action against a licensed healthcare provider arising out of the matters that are the subject of evaluation and review by such committee. No person who was in attendance at a meeting of such committee shall be permitted or required to testify in any such civil action about any evidence or other matters produced or presented during the proceedings of such committee or about any findings, recommendations, evaluations, opinions, or other actions of such committee or any members thereof, except that information, documents, or records otherwise available from original sources are not to be construed as immune from discovery or use in any such civil action merely because they were presented during proceedings of such committee.

Any documents or records that have been presented to the review committee by any witness shall be returned to the witness, if requested by him or her or if ordered to be produced by a court in any action, with copies thereof to be retained by the committee at its discretion. Nothing in this law shall prohibit a court of record, after a hearing and for good cause arising from extraordinary circumstances being shown, from ordering the disclosure of such proceedings, minutes, records, reports, or communications (Nebraska Revised Statutes § 25-12,123).

Section 71-2048 specifies that the proceedings, minutes, records, and reports of any medical staff committee or utilization review committee, together with all communications originating in such committees, are privileged communications that may not be disclosed or obtained by legal discovery proceedings unless:

- The privilege is waived by the patient.

- A court of record, after a hearing and for good cause arising from extraordinary circumstances being shown, orders the disclosure of such proceedings, minutes, records, reports, or communications.

Nothing in the peer review statutes shall be construed as providing any privilege to hospital medical records kept with respect to any patient in the ordinary course of business of operating a hospital nor to any facts or information contained in such records, nor shall those laws preclude or affect discovery of or production of evidence relating to hospitalization or treatment of any patient in the ordinary course of hospitalization of such patient.

Nevada

Nevada Revised Statutes § 49.265 states that except as otherwise provided, the proceedings and records of:

- Organized committees of hospitals and organizations that provide emergency medical services, having the responsibility of evaluation and improvement of the quality of care rendered by those hospitals or organizations and review committees of medical or dental societies are not subject to discovery proceedings.

New Hampshire

Records of a hospital committee organized to evaluate the care and treatment of patients or to reduce morbidity and mortality and testimony by hospital trustees, medical staff, employees, or other committee attendees relating to activities of the quality assurance committee are confidential and privileged. The facility must protect them from direct or indirect means of discovery, subpoena, or admission into evidence in any judicial or administrative proceeding, except that in the case of a legal action brought by a quality assurance committee to revoke or restrict a physician's license or hospital staff privileges, or in a proceeding alleging repetitive malicious action and personal injury brought against a physician, a committee's records are discoverable (New Hampshire Statutes § 151:13-a).

New Jersey

Under New Jersey Statutes § 2A:84A-22.8, information and data secured by and in the possession of a utilization review committee established by any certified hospital or extended care facility in the performance of its duties shall not be revealed or disclosed in any manner or under any circumstances by any member of such committee except to:

- A patient's attending physician.
- The chief administrative officer of the hospital or extended care facility that it serves.
- The medical executive committee, or comparable enforcement unit, of such hospital or extended care facility.
- Representatives of, including intermediaries or carriers for, government agencies in the performance of their duties, under the provisions of federal and state law.
- Any hospital service corporation, medical service corporation, or insurance company with which said patient has pertinent coverage under a contract, policy or certificate, the terms of which authorize the carrier to request and be given such information and data.

New Mexico

New Mexico Statutes § 41-9-5 provides for confidentiality of records of review organizations. All data and information acquired by a review organization in the exercise of its duties and functions shall be held in confidence and shall not be disclosed to anyone except to the extent necessary to carry out one or more of the purposes of the review organization or in a judicial appeal from the action of a review organization. No person described shall disclose what transpired at a meeting of a review organization except to the extent necessary to carry out one or more of the purposes of a review organization or in a judicial appeal from the action of a review organization. Information, documents, or records otherwise available from original sources shall not be immune from discovery or use in any civil action merely because they were presented during proceedings of a review organization.

Any disclosure other than that authorized by the Review Organization Immunity Act of data and information acquired by a review organization or of what transpired at a review organization meeting is guilty of a petty misdemeanor and shall be punished by imprisonment for not to exceed six months or by a fine of not more than $100, or both (*Id.* § 41-9-6).

New York

No person in attendance at a meeting when a medical or a quality assurance review or a medical and dental malpractice prevention program or an incident-reporting function described herein was performed, shall be required to testify about what transpired during the meeting. The prohibition relating to discovery of testimony shall not apply to the statements made by any person in attendance at such a meeting who is a party to an action or proceeding concerning the subject matter that was reviewed at such meeting (New York Education Law § 6527).

North Carolina

The proceedings of a medical review committee, the records and materials it produces, and the materials it considers shall be confidential and not considered public records, and shall not be subject to discovery or introduction into evidence in any civil action against a hospital or a provider of professional health services that results from matters that are the subject of evaluation and review by the committee (General Statutes of North Carolina § 131E-95).

North Dakota

North Dakota Century Code § 23-01-02.1 provides that any information, data, reports, or records made available to a mandatory hospital committee or facility committee as required by state or federal law or by the Joint Commission on Accreditation of Healthcare Organizations by a hospital or extended care facility or any physician or surgeon or group of physicians or surgeons operating a clinic or outpatient care facility in this state or to an internal quality assurance review committee of any hospital or extended care facility in this state are confidential and may be used by such committees and the members thereof only in the exercise of the proper functions of the committees. The proceedings and records of such a committee are not subject to subpoena or discovery or introduction into evidence in any civil action arising out of any matter subject to consideration by the committee. Information, documents, or records otherwise available from original sources are not immune from discovery or use in any civil action merely because they were presented during the proceedings of such a committee.

Ohio

Any information, data, reports, or records made available to a quality assurance committee or utilization committee of a hospital or of any not-for-profit healthcare corporation that is a member of the hospital or of which the hospital is a member shall be confidential and shall be used by the committee and the committee members only in the exercise of the proper functions of the committee. Any information, data, reports, or records made available to a utilization committee of a state or local medical society composed of doctors of medicine or doctors of osteopathic medicine and surgery shall be confidential and shall be used by the committee and the committee members only in the exercise of the proper functions of the committee.

A right of action similar to that a patient may have against an attending physician for misuse of information, data, reports, or records arising out of the physician-patient relationship, shall accrue against a member of a quality assurance committee or utilization committee for misuse of any information, data, reports, or records furnished to the committee by an attending physician. Information, data, or reports furnished to a utilization committee of a state or local medical society shall contain no name of any person involved therein (Ohio Revised Code § 2305.24).

Section 2305.251 of the Ohio Code provides for confidentiality of information of utilization review committees.

Oklahoma

Recipients of peer and utilization review information shall use or publish such information, interviews, reports, statements, memoranda, or other data relating to the condition and treatment of any person only for the purpose of advancing medical research or medical education in the interest of reducing morbidity or mortality, except that a summary of such studies may be released by any such group for general publication. In all events, the identity of any person whose condition or treatment has been studied shall be confidential and shall not be revealed under any circumstances. Any information furnished shall not contain the name of the person upon whom information is furnished and shall not violate the confidential relationship of patient and doctor. All information, interviews, reports, statements, memoranda, or other data furnished by reason of this statute, and any findings or conclusions resulting from such studies, are declared to be privileged communications that may not be used or offered or received in evidence in any legal proceeding of any kind or character. Any attempt to use or offer any such information, interviews, reports, statements, memoranda, or other data, findings or conclusions, or any part thereof, unless waived by the interested parties, shall constitute prejudicial error in any such proceeding (63 Oklahoma Statutes § 1-1709).

Oregon

Oregon Revised Statutes § 41.675 provides for the inadmissibility of certain healthcare facility and training data. Under this statute, *data* means written reports, notes, or records of tissue committees, governing bodies, or committees of a licensed healthcare facility; and medical staff committees and similar committees of professional societies in connection either with training, supervision, or discipline of physicians or with the grant, denial, restriction, or termination of clinical privileges at a healthcare facility. The term also includes the written reports, notes, or records of utilization review and peer review organizations.

All data shall be privileged and shall not be admissible in evidence in any judicial proceeding, but this privilege does not affect the admissibility in evidence of a party's medical records dealing with a party's hospital care and treatment.

Pennsylvania

According to Pennsylvania Statutes § 425.4, the proceedings and records of a review committee shall be held in confidence and shall not be subject to discovery or introduction into evidence in any civil action against a professional healthcare provider arising out of the matters that are the subject of evaluation and review by such committee, and no person who was in attendance at a meeting of such committee shall be permitted or required to testify in any such civil action about any evidence or other matters produced or presented during the proceedings of such committee or about any findings, recommendations, evaluations, opinions, or other actions of such committee or any members thereof. However, information, documents, or records otherwise available from original sources are not immune from discovery or use in any such civil action merely because they were presented during proceedings of such committee.

Rhode Island

General Laws of Rhode Island § 5-37.3-7 governing medical peer review committees permits healthcare providers to make confidential healthcare information available to medical peer review committees without authorization. Confidential healthcare information before a medical peer review committee shall remain strictly confidential, and any person found guilty of the unlawful disclosure of that information shall be subject to the penalties provided in this chapter. Except as otherwise provided, the proceedings and records of medical peer review committees shall not be subject to discovery or introduction into evidence.

South Carolina

Code of Laws of South Carolina § 40-71-20 provides that all proceedings of and all data and information acquired by peer review committees in the exercise of their duties are confidential unless a respondent in proceeding requests in writing that they be made public. These proceedings and documents are not subject to discovery, subpoena, or introduction into evidence in any civil action except upon appeal from the committee action. Information, documents, or records that are otherwise available from original sources are not immune from discovery or use in a civil action merely because they were presented during the committee proceedings, nor shall any complainant or witness before the committee be prevented from testifying in a civil action about matters of which he or she has knowledge apart from the committee proceedings or revealing such matters to third persons.

South Dakota

The proceedings, records, reports, statements, minutes, or any other data whatsoever, of any peer review committee, or any administrative or medical committee, department, section, board of directors, or audit group, including the medical audit committee of a licensed hospital, relating to the quality, type, or necessity of care rendered by a member of a hospital medical staff or by hospital personnel, or acquired in the evaluation of the competency, character, experience, or performance of a physician, dentist, or allied health professional seeking admission or reappointment to the medical staff of a hospital, shall not be subject to discovery or disclosure and shall not be admissible as evidence in any action of any kind in any court or arbitration forum. However, the prohibition relating to discovery of evidence does not apply to deny a physician access to or use of information upon which a decision regarding his or her staff privileges was based. The prohibition relating to discovery of evidence does not apply to deny any person or his or her counsel in the defense of an action against him or her access to the materials covered under this section (South Dakota Codified Laws § 36-4-26.1).

Tennessee

All information, interviews, incident or other reports, statements, memoranda, or other data furnished to any medical review or peer review committee and any findings, conclusions, or recommendations resulting from the proceedings of such committee are privileged. The records and proceedings of any such committees are confidential and shall be used by such committee and the members thereof only in the exercise of the proper functions of the committee. The records and proceedings shall not be public records nor be available for court subpoena or for discovery proceedings. One proper function of such committees shall include advocacy for physicians before other medical peer review committees, peer review organizations, healthcare entities, private and governmental insurance carriers, national or local accreditation bodies, and the state Board of Medical Examiners of this or any other state. The disclosure of confidential, privileged peer review committee information to such entities during advocacy, as a report to the board of medical examiners under, or to the affected physician under review does not constitute either a waiver of confidentiality or privilege.

Nothing contained in this statute applies to records made in the regular course of business by a hospital or other provider of health care. Information, documents, or records otherwise available from original sources are not to be construed as immune from discovery or use in any civil proceedings merely because they were presented during proceedings of such committee (Tennessee Code Annotated § 63-6-219).

Texas

Under the Texas Health and Safety Code § 161.032, the records and proceedings of a medical committee are confidential and are not subject to court subpoena. The records and proceedings may be used by the committee and the committee members only in the exercise of proper committee functions. This law does not apply to records made or maintained in the regular course of business by a hospital, health maintenance organization, or extended care facility.

Texas Revised Civil Statute article 4495b, the Practice Act, provides that except as otherwise provided in the act, all proceedings and records of a medical peer review committee are confidential, and all communications made to a medical peer review committee are privileged. If a judge makes a preliminary finding that such proceedings, records, or communications are relevant to an anticompetitive action, or a civil rights proceeding, then such proceedings, records, or communications are not confidential to the extent they are deemed relevant.

Disclosure of confidential peer review committee information to the affected physician pertinent to the matter under review shall not constitute waiver of the confidentiality provisions provided in this act. If a medical peer review committee takes action that could result in censure, suspension, restriction, limitation, revocation, or denial of membership or privileges in a health-care entity, the affected physician shall be provided a written copy of the recommendation of the medical peer review committee and a copy of the final decision, including a statement of the basis for the decision *(Id.)*.

Unless disclosure is required or authorized by law, records or determinations of or communications to a medical peer review committee are not subject to subpoena or discovery and are not admissible as evidence in any civil judicial or administrative proceeding without waiver of the privilege of confidentiality executed in writing by the committee.

Utah

The Department of Human Services, the Division of Mental Health within the Department of Human Services, scientific and healthcare research organizations affiliated with institutions of higher education, the Utah State Medical Association or any of its allied medical societies, peer review committees, professional review organizations, professional societies and associations, or any health facility's in-house staff committee may only use or publish the material received or gathered for the purpose of advancing medical research or medical education in the interest of reducing morbidity or mortality, except that a summary of studies conducted in accordance with Section 26-25-1 may be released by those groups for general publication (Utah Statutes § 26-25-2).

All information, including information required for the medical and health section of birth certificates as determined by the state registrar of vital records, interviews, reports, statements, memoranda, or other data furnished by reason of the Health Code's confidential information chapter and any findings or conclusions resulting from those studies are privileged communications and may not be used or received in evidence in any legal proceeding of any kind or character (*Id.* § 26-25-3).

Under § 58-12-43, information relating to the adequacy of quality of medical care provided to state or hospital boards is confidential.

Vermont

The proceedings, reports, and records of peer review are confidential and privileged, and shall not be subject to discovery or introduction into evidence in any civil action against a provider of professional health services arising out of the matters that are subject to evaluation and review by such committee, and no person who was in attendance at a meeting of such committee shall be permitted or required to testify in any such civil action about any findings, recommendations, evaluations, opinions, or other actions of such committees or any members thereof. However, information, documents, or records otherwise available from original sources are not to be construed as immune from discovery or use in any such action merely because they were presented during the proceedings of such committee (26 Vermont Statutes Annotated § 1443).

Virginia

The proceedings, minutes, records, and reports of any medical staff committee, utilization review committee, or other committee, together with all communications, both oral and written, originating in or provided to such committees are privileged communications that may not be disclosed or obtained by legal discovery proceedings unless a circuit court, after a hearing and for good cause arising from extraordinary circumstances being shown, orders the disclosure of such proceedings, minutes, records, reports, or communications. Nothing in this statute, however, provides any privilege to hospital medical records kept with respect to any patient in the ordinary course of business of operating a hospital nor to any facts or information contained in such records, nor shall this statute preclude or affect discovery of or production of evidence relating to hospitalization or treatment of any patient in the ordinary course of hospitalization of such patient (Virginia Code § 8.01-581.17).

Private review agents must ensure that patient-specific medical records and information are kept strictly confidential except as authorized by the patient or by regulations (*Id.* § 38.2-5302).

Investigative information acquired by the Department of Health Professions' medical complaint investigative complaint committee or the

Board of Medicine in connection with possible disciplinary proceedings is confidential (*Id.* § 54.1-2910).

Washington

The proceedings, reports, and written records of a regularly constituted committee or board of a hospital whose duty it is to review and evaluate the quality of patient care, or of a member, employee, staffperson, or investigator of such a committee or board, shall not be subject to subpoena or discovery proceedings in any civil action, except actions arising out of the recommendations of such committees or boards involving the restriction or revocation of the clinical or staff privileges of a healthcare provider (Revised Code of Washington § 4.24.250).

West Virginia

West Virginia Code § 30-3C-3 provides for confidentiality of review organization records. The proceedings and records of a review organization are confidential and privileged and shall not be subject to subpoena or discovery proceedings or be admitted as evidence in any civil action arising out of the matters that are subject to evaluation and review by such organization. However, information, documents, or records otherwise available from original sources are not immune from discovery or use in any civil action merely because they were presented during proceedings of such organization.

Wisconsin

Wisconsin Statutes § 146.38 provides that no person who participates in the review or evaluation of the services of healthcare providers or facilities or charges for such services may disclose any information acquired in connection with such review or evaluation except as provided in the statutes.

All organizations or evaluators reviewing or evaluating the services of healthcare providers shall keep a record of their investigations, inquiries, proceedings, and conclusions. No such record may be released to any person except as provided in the statutes. No such record may be used in any civil action for personal injuries against the healthcare provider or facility. However, information, documents, or records presented during the review or evaluation are not immune from discovery or use in any civil action merely because they were so presented.

Information acquired in connection with the review and evaluation of healthcare services shall be disclosed, and records of such review and evaluation shall be released, with the identity of any patient whose treatment is reviewed being withheld unless the patient has granted permission to disclose identity, in the following circumstances:

- To the healthcare provider or facility whose services are being reviewed or evaluated, upon the request of such provider or facility.

- To any person with the consent of the healthcare provider or facility whose services are being reviewed or evaluated.

- To the person requesting the review or evaluation, for use solely for the purpose of improving the quality of health care, avoiding the improper utilization of the services of healthcare providers and facilities, and determining the reasonable charges for such services.

- In a report in statistical form; which may identify any provider or facility to which the statistics relate.

- With regard to an action under § 895.70, to a court of record after issuance of a subpoena.

- With regard to any criminal matter, to a court of record, and after issuance of a subpoena.

- To the appropriate examining or licensing board or agency, when the organization or evaluator conducting the review or evaluation determines that such action is advisable.

Any person who discloses information or releases a record in violation of this section, other than through a good faith mistake, is civilly liable therefor to any person harmed by the disclosure or release.

Wyoming

Wyoming Statute § 35-17-105 provides that information of review organizations must be confidential and privileged. All reports, findings, proceedings, and data of the professional standard review organizations are confidential and privileged, and are not subject to discovery or introduction into evidence in any civil action. However, information, documents, or other records otherwise available from original sources are not to be construed as immune from discovery or use in any civil action merely because they were presented during proceedings of the organization.

Wyoming Statute § 35-2-602 makes all reports, findings, proceedings, and data of hospital medical staff committees privileged and confidential.

Conclusion

As this chapter illustrates, peer review statutes vary from state to state. Thus, to determine the degree of confidentiality of the peer review activities of a healthcare facility, the facility's attorneys must review both the federal and state statutes and court decisions. In addition, state regulations as of the public health department or similar agency may provide for confidentiality. And any healthcare facility should have in place safeguards that guard such information from inadvertent disclosure. Comprehensive state confidentiality protection does little good if peer review information becomes common knowledge.

Endnotes

1. *Beddice v. Doctors Hospital,* 50 F.R.D. 249 (D. D.C. 1970).

2. *Matchett v. Superior Court,* 40 Cal. Rptr. 317 (1974). See generally William Morton, "Are You Protected by the Peer Review Privilege?" *Legal Aspects of Medical Practice* 16, No. 8 (August 1988), pp. 1, 8.

3. 42 USC § 11137(b).

4. 42 CFR § 476.141. *See generally* Theodore LeBlang and W. Eugene Basanta, *The Law of Medical Practice in Illinois* (1986), p. 95.

5. Nebraska Revised Statutes § 71-2048 (1986). *See generally* Christopher Morter, "The Health Care Quality Improvement Act of 1986: Will Physicians Find Peer Review More Inviting?" *Virginia Law* Review 74 (September 1988), pp. 1115, 1132-34.

6. Idaho Code § 39-1392b (1987).

7. American Medical Association, *A Compendium of State Peer Immunity Laws* (Chicago: AMA, 1988), p. viii.

8. Christopher Morter, "The Health Care Quality Improvement Act of 1986: Will Physicians Find Peer Review More Inviting?" *Virginia Law Review* 74 (September 1988), pp. 1115, 1132-33.

9. Alaska Statutes § 18.23.030 (1991).

7

Exceptions to Confidentiality

Introduction

Although medical records and other healthcare information are confidential and, as discussed in Chapter 4, some have increased confidentiality protection, this type of information does little good if no one can use it. Thus, the law provides for a number of exceptions to the confidentiality rules so that providers and others can use this information when necessary. The most usual exception is for medical diagnosis and treatment and related administrative matters, including billing. Other exceptions include communicable disease reporting; reporting of potential danger from a patient; criminal reporting such as child or elder abuse, attempt to obtain drugs illegally, or Medicare fraud; disclosure for research and medical education; disclosure for statistical purposes; disclosure for licensing, regulation, or accreditation; and disclosure pursuant to court order.

Disclosure for Diagnosis, Treatment, and Related Administrative Matters

Confidentiality statutes and regulations often provide for the disclosure of medical information among providers for the purposes of diagnosis and treatment. For example, Oklahoma Statutes Title 43A, § 1-109, after noting that medical records are confidential, specifies that such information is available only to persons or agencies actively engaged in patient treatment or related administrative work. Florida specifies that even without patient consent, a hospital may disclose its patients' records to:

- Hospital personnel for use in connection with treatment of patients.

- Hospital personnel only for internal hospital administrative purposes associated with payment.

- The Hospital Cost Containment Board [Florida Administrative Code r. 59A-3.158(3)].

Even if such a statute does not have an express authorization for disclosure of medical information as necessary for diagnosis and treatment, such an exception to the general confidentiality of medical information is implied. Courts have consistently found that patients have consented to the release of medical information as necessary for diagnosis and treatment. As one medical records expert puts it:

> When patients request care from an institution, it is logical to assume that they are also voluntarily agreeing to the disclosure of information to those professionals directly involved in furnishing such care. Knowledge of what others are doing or have done for a patient, reactions to present and past treatment, patient progress, recommendations concerning treatment changes, and plans for follow-up care are examples of specific information essential to an understanding of current patient needs. Use of institutional patient-identifiable information for current care purposes, therefore, does not require specific patient authorization.[1]

The facility should have a policy identifying staff members with patient care responsibilities, and the degree of access to patient records each should have as well as security measures to prevent unauthorized access.[2]

Disclosure for Billing

In today's managed care environment, providers must disclose medical re-cord information for billing purposes. Access to this information is neces-sary to substantiate insurance claims. The law provides for disclosure of confidential patient-identifiable medical information for billing purposes in two ways: by providing for patient consent in the third-party payment con-tract or by a statute or regulation authorizing such disclosure. Maryland Health-General Code § 4-305 provides that healthcare providers may dis-close medical records without patient authorization to third-party payers and their agents or any other person obligated by contract or law to pay for the health care rendered for the sole purposes of:

- Submitting a bill to the third-party payer.

- Reasonable prospective, concurrent, or retrospective utilization re-view or predetermination of benefit coverage.

- Review, audit, and investigation of a specific claim for payment of benefits.

- Coordinating benefit payments under more than one sickness and accident, dental, or hospital and medical insurance policy.

Texas Revised Civil Statute article 4495b allows providers to disclose those parts of medical records reflecting charges and specific services ren-dered when necessary in collection of fees for medical services provided by physicians, professional associations, or other entities qualified to render or arrange for medical services. This statute also provides for disclosure to individuals, corporations, or government agencies involved in the payment or collection of fees for medical services rendered by physicians.

Under such contracts or statutes, providers should only disclose the medical information necessary to accomplish the billing or related purpose and seek patient consent for any further disclosures.

Communicable Disease Reporting

Almost all jurisdictions require reporting of certain sexually transmitted or communicable diseases to a government agency, typically the health de-partment, for purposes of disease prevention and control. Statutes and regulations providing for such reporting typically limit further disclosure of patient-identifiable information. Among common reportable diseases are:

- Tuberculosis.
- Sexually transmitted diseases, including syphilis, gonorrhea, and AIDS.
- Cancer.
- Sentinel birth defects.
- Occupational diseases.
- Hepatitis.
- Botulism.
- Cholera.
- Plague.
- Smallpox.
- Typhus.
- Yellow fever.

In Tennessee, for example, every physician or other person who diagnoses, treats, or prescribes for a sexually transmitted disease and every superintendent or manager of a clinic, hospital, laboratory, or penal institution must report the case to those agencies as directed by the commissioner of health and environment (Tennessee Code § 68-10-101). All records and information held by the Department of Health and Environment or a local health department concerning sexually transmitted diseases are confidential and may not be released except as follows:

- To medical personnel, appropriate state agencies, or county and district courts to enforce the laws governing control and treatment of sexually transmitted diseases.
- In cases involving minors, only the name, age, address and sexually transmitted disease, to the appropriate agencies under the Tennessee Child Abuse law.[3]
- When ordered by a trial court judge who finds each of the following:
  - The information is material, relevant, and reasonably calculated to be admissible evidence during legal proceedings.
  - The probative value of the evidence[4] outweighs the subject's and the public's interest in maintaining its confidentiality.
  - The litigation cannot be resolved without disclosure.

- The evidence is necessary in order to avoid substantial injustice to the party seeking it and either disclosure would result in no significant harm to the person examined or treated, or it would be substantially unfair as between the requesting party and the person who is examined or treated not to require disclosure (*Id.* § 68-10-113).

State statutes and regulations often provide for a penalty for failure to make required reports. However, they often also provide a penalty for breaches of the required confidentiality if the confidential report is improperly disclosed. Some jurisdictions require any disclosure of sexually transmitted disease or similar information to be accompanied by a warning. In Washington state, for example, every disclosure of sexually transmitted disease test results other than to the subject of the test or his or her representative or among providers to provide healthcare services must be accompanied by a written statement as follows:

This information has been disclosed to you from records whose confidentiality is protected by state law. State law prohibits you from making any future disclosure of it without the specific written consent of the person to whom it pertains. A general authorization for the release of medical or other information is NOT sufficient for this purpose [Washington Revised Code § 70.25.105(5)].

For a complete discussion of state reporting laws, see Tomes, *Healthcare Records Management, Disclosure, and Retention: The Complete Legal Guide* (Chicago: Probus Publishing Co., 1993, pp. 362-93).

Reporting of Danger from Patients

In certain circumstances, providers can breach the physician-patient or similar privileges and/or violate the confidentiality of medical records to protect others endangered by the patient. The most famous case finding that healthcare professionals had a duty to warn those who could be foreseeably injured by their patients arose in the context of a psychotherapist-client relationship. In *Tarasoff v. Regents of the University of California*,[5] the California Supreme Court held that a therapist treating a mentally ill patient owes a duty of reasonable care to warn threatened third parties against foreseeable danger inherent in the patient's condition. In this case, a patient had made explicit threats toward his former girlfriend during therapy. The therapist failed to warn the girlfriend and the patient eventually killed her.

Courts have expanded this duty to other areas, primarily involving communicable diseases and the side-effects of medications. Courts have found physicians liable to third parties for failure to warn about the possibility of contracting scarlet fever from the patient, the possibility of infection from the patient's wounds, the possibility of contracting smallpox, and for driving while under the influence of medication.[6]

Some states have statutes authorizing disclosure of medical information without patient consent in cases involving threats to others or the commission of a crime. In addition to other grounds for disclosure, Rhode Island provides that confidential healthcare information may be disclosed to law enforcement personnel if someone is in danger from the patient, if the patient tries to get narcotics from the healthcare provider illegally, and in gunshot wound cases [Rhode Island General Laws § 5-37.3-4(b)].

The most complicated legal issues involve whether a practitioner should warn the spouse or other sexual partner of a patient with AIDS or who is HIV-infected about the possibility of contracting the disease. The issue is more complicated than in other communicable or even sexually transmitted disease cases because of the special stigma attached to AIDS and because, unlike tuberculosis, for example, it cannot be spread through casual contact. However, the disease's incurable nature may require a warning of those foreseeably at risk, even though the disease is not easy to transmit. On the other hand, notifying sexual partners or others may actually harm efforts to prevent the spread of AIDS by deterring those who may be infected from coming forward for testing. And, as discussed in Chapter 4, virtually every state has enhanced protection for the confidentiality of AIDS/HIV information, with severe sanctions for wrongful disclosure of such information.

Some states, however, do provide for disclosure to protect others—either to the Department of Health or similar agencies, or to someone threatened by the patient if a court orders the disclosure. In New Jersey, for example, providers may relapse AIDS or HIV-infection records, without patient consent, to the Department of Health as required by state or federal law and as permitted by rules and regulations adopted by the commissioner of health for purposes of disease prevention and control. The state must keep the patient's identity confidential and may only use the information for research and study purposes (New Jersey Revised Statute § 26:5C-8). In addition, healthcare providers may disclose such information if a court so orders after finding good cause for the disclosure. In determining whether good cause exists, the court must weigh the public interest and the need for disclosure against the injury to the person who is the subject of the record, to the physician-patient relationship, and to the services offered by the testing program. If the court authorizes disclosure, it must impose appropriate safeguards against unauthorized disclosure (*Id.* § 26:5C-9).

Of course, healthcare professionals may counsel HIV-infected patients how to protect others and suggest that they tell their sexual or needle-sharing partners to get testing, counseling, or treatment, as appropriate. As to warning others, the American Medical Association position provides a good starting point for considering the issue:

> Where there is no statute that mandates or prohibits reporting of seropositive individuals to public health authorities and it is clear that the seropositive individual is endangering an identified third party, the physician should (1) attempt to persuade the infected individual to cease endangering the third party; (2) if persuasion fails, notify authorities; and (3) if authorities take no action, notify and counsel the endangered third party.[7]

New York law follows this guidance as permits the physician to disclose HIV information to those in significant risk of infection if the infected person will not do so after counseling the infected person and warning him or her of the intention to disclose. However, under this statute, the physician cannot reveal the name of the infected person. The physician cannot be held liable for disclosing or failing to disclose this information (New York Public Health Law § 2782).

Obviously, the advice of a healthcare attorney is a must before warning anyone of a patient's HIV status. And a prudent healthcare professional should seek legal counsel before breaching confidentiality in *any* situation in which a third party is endangered other than simply following a statutory or regulatory duty to report to the health department or similar agency. See Chapter 4's recitation of confidentiality laws for communicable and sexually transmitted diseases.

Crime Reporting

The law often provides for an exception to the physician-patient privilege or to the general confidentiality of medical records in criminal cases, particularly in cases of child or similar forms of abuse, such as elder abuse. These statutes typically require reporting of actual or suspected abuse and protect the person making the report from any liability for making the report as long as he or she made the report in good faith. Failure to make a required abuse report often subjects the healthcare provider to a criminal penalty and/or liability for any further injuries the child or other victim suffers because the abuse was allowed to continue.

In Arkansas, for example, any physician or other healthcare provider engaged in the admission, examination, care, or treatment who has reasonable cause to suspect that a child has been subjected to abuse, sexual abuse, or neglect or observes the child being subjected to conditions that would reasonably result in such abuse, must immediately report the abuse to the Department of Human Services. The provider may make the report directly to the department or make the report to the person in charge of the medical institution, who is then responsible for making the report to the department. The reporter must make the report immediately by telephone, then follow up with a written report within 48 hours if the department so requests. Anyone making such a report in good faith is immune from any liability for so doing, but failure to report subjects the offender to a $100 fine, up to five days in jail, and to civil liability for damages caused by failing to report. The same penalties apply in cases of false reports (Arkansas Statutes §§ 12-12-503 and following). Arkansas law also provides the physician-patient privilege does not apply to abuse cases (*Id.* § 12-12-511), so physicians may report abuse and testify about it without violating the privilege.

Many states have similar reporting requirements for elder abuse. In Missouri, for example, providers must report cases of abuse or neglect of residents of convalescent, nursing, and boarding homes (Missouri Revised Statutes § 198.070).

Some states require providers to report various crimes, notwithstanding the confidentiality of medical information. Rhode Island, for example, requires providers to report criminal or civil wrong doing in connection with Medicaid fraud to the Medicaid fraud control unit of the attorney general's office [Rhode Island General Laws § 5-37.3-4(b)]. The California Penal Code requires release of medical information if reason exists to believe that a crime was committed by or against a patient [California Penal Code § 1543(a)].

Disclosure for Research or Medical Education

As noted in Chapter 5, all jurisdictions allow access to medical records for research purposes but typically require researchers to refrain from disclosing patients' identities in reports. Medical information can also be disclosed to medical students, interns, student nurses, and others as necessary for medical education. Rhode Island, for example, authorizes disclosure of confidential medical information, without patient consent, for education and training within the same healthcare facility [Rhode Island General Laws § 5-37.3-4(b)]. Of course, such disclosure should be limited to legitimate research or educational needs, and those receiving such information should not redisclose it except as authorized by law. Prudence may dictate obtaining patient consent for such disclosures even when the law appears to permit disclosure without patient consent.

Disclosure for Statistical Purposes

Virtually all jurisdictions permit disclosure of medical information to the government for statistical reporting, such as reporting births and deaths to the appropriate state agency. States use such information to determine the need for federal and state health programs. For example, Montana Revised Statutes § 71-610, in conjunction with Nebraska Administrative Rules and Regulations 175-9-003.048, requires maternity homes and lying-in hospitals to report to the Department of Health on the first day of each month, the sex and date of birth of all children born in their respective institutions during the preceding month. The reports also show the names and addresses of the parents and the attending physician. Each facility must also file a birth certificate with the registrar of births within five days after the birth.

Disclosure for Licensing, Regulation, or Accreditation

In addition to other authorized disclosure, the law permits providers to release medical record information to licensing, regulatory, and accrediting authorities, such as health departments, the Joint Commission on Accreditation of Healthcare Organizations, and the like, even without patient consent, so these organizations can carry out their functions of ensuring quality patient care by their review of the institution's services. Of course, the institution, in releasing such information as is necessary for the inspection or other review of its operations, should only release necessary records and protect patient privacy as much as possible.

In Texas, for example, among other grounds for disclosure are:

- When, in license revocation proceedings, a patient is the complaining witness and disclosure is relevant to the claims or to the physician's defense.

- In disciplinary investigations or proceedings against a physician, provided the disciplinary board protects the identity of the patient.

Statutes often give health departments the authority to subpoena medical records for use in licensing determinations. In Maryland, for example, professional licensing and disciplinary boards may subpoena medical records for an investigation concerning licensure, certification, or discipline of a health professional or into the improper practice of a health profession [Maryland Health-General Code § 4-306(a)(2)].

Disclosure Pursuant to Court Order

All jurisdictions provide for disclosure of medical record information by subpoena or court order, either under a specific statute governing medical records or under their general subpoena statute, subject of course to any heightened confidentiality requirements. A *subpoena* is a court order compelling a witness to testify. A *subpoena duces tecum* is a court order compelling a witness to bring specified documents to the court. Under Mississippi's code, which is similar to that of many states, when a subpoena requires production of hospital records, the records custodian may comply by filing with the court clerk or the official or entity issuing the subpoena, a true and correct copy of the records described in the subpoena. The custodian must enclose the records in an inner envelope or wrapper, seal it, label the wrapper with the title and number of the case, the name of the witness, and the date of the subpoena, and enclose it in an outer envelope. The custodian must enclose an affidavit stating that he or she is the custodian and has the authority to certify the records, that the copy is a true copy of the records described in the subpoena, and that the records were prepared by hospital personnel in the ordinary course of business at or near the time of the act, condition, or event reported in the records. The custodian must also specify the amount of the reasonable charges for furnishing the record (Mississippi Code §§ 41-9-105, 41-9-109).

Because other statutes that provide for heightened confidentiality for certain types of medical information, such as AIDS/HIV status, and privileges, such as the physician-patient privilege, may affect whether medical records are subject to subpoena, providers should get legal advice before responding to the subpoena. See Tomes, *Healthcare Records Management, Disclosure and Retention: The Complete Legal Guide* (Chicago: Probus Publishing Co., 1993, pp. 394-417) for a discussion of each state's laws governing court-ordered disclosure of medical records.

Conclusion

Even though providers are authorized to disclose medical information for a number of uses, including patient care; billing; communicable disease reporting; reporting of threats to others; reporting of criminal acts; medical research and education; statistical purposes; licensing, regulation, and accreditation; and pursuant to a court order, the disclosure should be no greater than necessary to accomplish the purpose of the disclosure. The provider should make every reasonable effort to protect patient confidentiality as much as possible considering the nature of the disclosure.

Endnotes

1.   Jo Anne Czecowski Bruce, RRA, *Privacy and Confidentiality of Health Care Information.* Chicago: American Hospital Publishing, Inc., 1984, p. 30.

2.   *Id.* at pp. 30-31.

3.   Tennessee Code § 37-1-403.

4.   That is, the evidence's tendency to prove a particular proposition.

5.   17 Cal.3d 425, 131 Cal.Rptr. 14, 551 P.2d 334 (1976).

6.   B. Furrow, S. Johnson, T. Jost, and R. Schwartz, *Health Law: Cases, Materials, and Problems,* 2d ed. St. Paul, Minn.: West Publishing Co., 1991, pp. 315-16.

7.   American Medical Association, *HIV Blood Test Counseling: A.M.A. Physician Guidelines.* Chicago: AMA, 1988.

8

Disclosure on Request

Introduction

Patients may waive their rights to privacy and confidentiality and in fact do so every time they consent to the release of confidential medical information to others. Issues inherent in the disclosure of medical information on the patient's or another's request include who "owns" the records; who besides the patient may request records; what procedure to follow upon receipt of a request, including what constitutes a proper request; and what happens if the provider fails to allow access to the records.

Who Owns Medical Records?

Patients often think that they own their records and thus have an ownership right to them. However, many states have statutes or administrative regulations that specify that the actual physical record is the property of the provider. Such statutes usually add, however, that the patient who is the subject of the record has the right to review the information contained in the record. Massachusetts General Laws chapter 111, § 70, for example, specifies that the facility has custody of the medical record, but the patient has a right to inspect it. A provider can rely on this statement of the law—that providers own the records, subject to the patients' rights to review the information contained in the record—even in states that do not have a specific statute saying so. For example, in *Cannell v. Medical & Surgical Clinic*,[1] an Illinois appeals court held that the nature of the physician-patient relationship required disclosure of medical data to the patient or to the patient's representative upon request, but that the physician need not turn over the physical record to the patient.

Who May Consent to the Release of Medical Information?

Most states have statutes or administrative records that provide for patients and others to have access to medical records on request. These laws range from specific ones, providing detailed requirements that the patient and the facility must follow, to simple statements that patients have access to their records. In the latter situation, the provider should adopt bylaws specifying the procedure for release of medical record information on request in keeping with the confidential nature of the information.

In Colorado, for example, Colorado Revised Statute § 25-1-801 allows patients in healthcare facilities or their designated representatives to inspect their records, other than those relating to psychiatric or psychological problems or those that an independent third-party psychiatrist believes would have a significant negative effect on the patient, at reasonable times and on reasonable notice. The patient or his or her representative is also entitled to a summary of his or her psychiatric or psychological problems following termination of the treatment program. Following the patient's discharge, he or she is entitled on submission of a written authorization/request for records,[2] and payment of reasonable costs, to have copies of his or her records, including X rays. Section 25-1-802 contains virtually identical language covering patient records in the custody of individual healthcare providers.

Most state laws permit the patient or the patient's physician or authorized attorney to examine and copy the patient's medical records. If the patient is deceased, the executor of the patient's estate is authorized to have access to the patient's medical records. Most states provide that requests to release medical information about minors or incompetent patients should be signed by their parents or legal guardians. One exception to this rule in many states is that if the minor is permitted by law to consent to the treatment that is recorded in the records,[2] the provider may disclose that portion of the records upon receiving the minor's consent without the signature of a parent or guardian.

In states that have statutes providing for healthcare powers of attorney, the person who has been appointed to make the patient's healthcare decisions can also consent to the disclosure of medical information for the patient.

Most jurisdictions permit physicians to deny patients access to their medical records if that access would be harmful to the patient. In Arkansas, for example, if a physician believes that a patient should be denied access to a medical record, for any reason, that physician must provide the patient or the patient's guardian or attorney with a written determination that disclosure of such information would be detrimental to the patient's health or well-being [Arkansas Code § 16-46-106(b)].

What Is the Procedure upon Receipt of a Request for Medical Records?

Some states specify an exact procedure for a provider who receives a request from a patient to examine or copy his or her medical records. Others simply specify the contents of a proper authorization for release of medical records. Still others leave it up to the institution to formulate a policy for the release of medical information on request.

Montana Code § 50-16-541 specifies that on receipt of a written request from a patient to examine or copy all or part of his or her medical records, a healthcare provider, as promptly as required under the circumstances, but no later than 10 days after receiving the request, must:

- Make the information available to the patient for examination during regular business hours or provide a copy, if requested, to the patient.
- Inform the patient if the information does not exist or cannot be found.
- Inform the patient and provide the name and address, if known, of the healthcare provider who maintains the record if the healthcare provider does not itself maintain the record.
- Deny the request in whole or in part and inform the patient.[3]

Sometimes a state statute or administrative regulations specify what composes a proper request for medical records. In Texas, for example, the written consent for medical information must include:

- The information or medical records to be covered by the release.

- The reasons or purposes for the release.

- The person to whom the information is to be released [Texas Revised Civil Statutes article 4495b, § 5.08(j)].

Often statutes provide more detailed guidelines for medical information with increased confidentiality protection (see Chapter 4). For example, in Illinois a written request for the disclosure of records of patients treated for alcohol or drug abuse must contain the:

- Specific name or general designation of the program or person permitted to make the disclosure.

- Name or title of the individual or name of the organization to which disclosure is to be made.

- Name of the patient.

- Identification of the specific information to be released.

- Reason for the release or disclosure.

- Date on which the consent is signed.

- Signature of the patient or the patient's representative if the patient is a minor or incompetent.

- A statement that the consent is subject to revocation at any time, except to the extent that the program or person who is to make the disclosure has already acted in reliance on the consent.

- Date, event, or condition on which the consent will expire, if not revoked [Illinois Administrative Code Title 77, § 2058.318(a)].

As to release of medical records generally, Illinois simply provides that hospitals should issue policies and procedures governing such release upon request [*Id.* § 250.1510(b)(5)].

When a statute or regulation does not specify the contents of a valid request, the written authorization for release of medical record information should contain at least the following:

- Name of the provider that is to release the information.

- Name of the individual or entity that is to receive the information.

- Patient's full name, address, and date of birth.

- Purpose of the disclosure.

- Extent or nature of the information to be released, with inclusive dates of treatment.

- Specific date, event, or condition upon which the authorization will expire unless the patient or his or her representative revokes it earlier.

- Statement that the patient or his or her representative can revoke the authorization except as to the release of information already released in good faith.

- Date the consent is signed.

- Signature of the patient or legal representative.[4]

The facility should have a policy specifying the preceding contents of a proper request, and specifying:

- Rretention of the authorization in the patient's medical records.

- Notation on the authorization or on the medical records showing what information was released, the date of release, and containing the signature of the releaser.[5]

- Prohibitions, if any, on redisclosure of the information.

The policy should also specify who may consent for minors or incompetent patients and what evidence is necessary to demonstrate legal authority to consent for the patient, such as a court order showing appointment as a guardian.

The provider should require a consent form signed by the patient or his or her legal representative or a subpoena before releasing medical information to the patient's attorney.

Sanctions for Failure to Provide Patients Access to Their Records

Often state statutes specify a period of time within which the healthcare professional or entity must provide copies of properly requested medical records. In Louisiana, for example, if the provider does not furnish the record within a reasonable time (defined as within 15 days following receipt of the request and written authorization for disclosure) and the patient has to obtain a court order or subpoena to get the record, the provider is liable for reasonable attorney fees and expenses incurred in obtaining the court order or subpoena (Louisiana Revised Statutes § 40:1299.96).

Other states make failure to comply with a patient's request for disclosure of medical information a ground for disciplinary action (see, for example, Minnesota Statutes § 147.091).

Conclusion

Patients can waive their rights to confidentiality of healthcare information and disclose the contents of their medical information for others. Providers need to ensure that the person consenting, if not the patient, has the legal authority to do so and need to have a proper disclosure policy to disclose the requested information in a timely manner to an authorized recipient in order not to be liable for failure to disclose the information.

Endnotes

1.   21 Ill. App. 3d 383, 315 N.R. 2d 278 (3d Dist. 1974).

2.   Many states permit minors to consent to treatment for pregnancy, sexually transmitted diseases, and alcohol and drug aburs. See Tomes, *Informed Consent: A Guide for the Healthcare Professional* (Chicago: Probus Publishing Co., 1993), p. 11.

3.   Under Montana law, the provider may deny a patient access to healthcare information if the provider reasonably concludes one of the following circumstances exists:

   • Knowledge of the healthcare information would be injurious to the health of the patient.

   • Knowledge of the healthcare information could reasonably be expected to lead to the patient's identification of an individual who provided information in confidence and under circumstances in which confidentiality was appropriate.

   • Knowledge of the healthcare information could reasonably be expected to cause danger to the life or safety of any individual.

   • Healthcare information was compiled and is used solely for litigation, quality assurance, peer review, or administrative purposes.

- Healthcare information may disclose birth out of wedlock or provide information from which birth out of wedlock might be obtained.

- The healthcare provider obtained information from a person other than the patient.

- Access to the healthcare information is otherwise prohibited by law (Montana Code § 50-16-542).

4.   Edna Huffman, *Medical Record Management* 9th ed. (Berwyn, Ill.: Physician's Record Co., 1990), p. 605.

5.   *Id.* at 605-606.

9

Confidentiality of Personal and Financial Information

Introduction

Although personal and financial information does not have as great a degree of protection as does medical information, providers must be aware that they should not disclose personal or financial information about a patient without having a proper purpose or the patient's consent to do so. After discussing the right to privacy about one's personal and financial affairs, Chapter 9 will specify what types of information a facility may release.

The Right to Confidentiality of Personal and Financial Information

The courts have only found a limited right to personal and financial privacy in the general federal constitutional right to privacy discussed in Chapter 1.[1] However, state constitutions may provide greater privacy protection than does the federal constitution, and many states have statutes providing some protection for such information. Illinois legislators, for example, passed the Insurance Information and Privacy Protection Act, which protects both medical record information and "personal information." Personal information consists of individually identifiable information gathered in connection with an insurance transaction from which judgments can be made about an individual's character, habits, avocations, finances, occupation, general reputation, credit, health, or any other personal characteristics, including an individual's name and address and medical record information. The statute sets out permissible disclosures and prohibits other disclosures. One who knowingly discloses information in violation of this act statute is subject to a monetary penalty of not more than $500 for each violation, not to exceed a total of $10,000 and is liable to the individual to whom the information relates for actual damages suffered (215 Illinois Compiled Statutes 5/1001 and following).

Many patient bills of rights also provide privacy protection for personal or financial information, in addition to medical information. The Connecticut Patients' Bill of Rights, for example, states that a patient has the right to "confidential treatment of his *personal* and medical records."[2]

Even absent a statute providing protection for nonmedical information, a court may find a provider liable for violating a patient's right to privacy for disclosing personal or financial information. The law recognizes several torts—civil wrongs—involving disclosure of private information, including invasion of privacy and public disclosure of private facts. For example, in one case,[3] the court found that a plastic surgeon who used "before-and-after" photographs of his patient's plastic surgery without her consent at a department store presentation and a television show promoting the presentation invaded her right to privacy. The court recognized that the right to privacy was not absolute, but noted that if there was any such right at all, it should include the right to obtain medical treatment without personal publicity.

In order to recover damages for an invasion of privacy, the plaintiff must establish one of the following:

- An intrusion upon his or her seclusion or solitude or into his or her private affairs.

- A public disclosure of embarrassing private facts.

- Publicity that places him or her in a false light in the public eye.

- An appropriation for the defendant's advantage, of the plaintiff's name or likeness.[4]

Some healthcare legal scholars have suggested that commercial use of body parts taken from patients may violate patients' rights to privacy on an invasion of privacy theory similar to the appropriation for the defendant's advantage of the plaintiff's name or likeness—but one of appropriation of the plaintiff's biological substances.[5] The genesis of this theory is the famous (or infamous) *Moore v. Regents of the University of California*[6] case. In this case the plaintiff sued his attending physician, the Regents of the University of California, who owned and operated the UCLA Medical Center, a university researcher, and Sandoz Pharmaceuticals Corporation for breach of his physician's duty to disclose a conflict of interest. The physician obtained informed consent to remove Moore's spleen after diagnosing hairy-cell leukemia but did not disclose that he had the researcher intended to conduct research upon the spleen for financial and competitive benefits. On follow-up visits, the physician obtained other tissue samples to be used in the research. The parties obtained patents on a cell line developed from Moore's T-lymphocytes and negotiated commercial agreements for development of the cell line and its products. In finding that the plaintiff had a valid claim, the Supreme Court of California noted that "a person of adult years and in sound mind has the right, in the exercise of control over his own body, to determine whether or not to submit to lawful medical treatment." The court held that a physician has a duty, in obtaining informed consent, to disclose all information material to the patient's decision, including personal interests unrelated to the patient's health, whether research or economic, that may affect the physician's medical judgment.

What Information Can a Provider Release About a Patient?

Of course, not all information about a patient is protected by confidentiality laws. Generally, a healthcare institution may release the following without patient authorization unless the patient has requested that the facility withhold the following information:

- Patient name.
- Date of admission.
- Condition description (for example, critical, serious, or stable).[7]

Of course, the law and common sense dictate that particularly when the patient's condition involves an area of particularly sensitive medical information, such as alcohol or drug abuse treatment or AIDS/HIV treatment, even disclosing that the patient has been hospitalized for that condition could violate his or her right to privacy. Similarly, even disclosing that a celebrity is a patient of the institution may violate the celebrity's rights to privacy. When in doubt about whether disclosure of personal or financial information is permissible, the provider should seek patient consent. Without such consent or a clear statutory or regulatory duty to disclose the information, the provider should not disclose it unless advised that the disclosure is proper by legal counsel.

Conclusion

Although the law does not protect personal and financial information as completely as it does medical information, providers should be aware that patient rights to privacy are not limited to medical information concerning them and not release personal or financial information without legal authority to do so and a proper reason for doing so.

Endnotes

1. See *Plante v. Gonzales*, 575 F.2d 1119 (1978).

2. Connecticut General Statute § 19a-550 (emphasis added).

3. *Vassiliades v. Garfinckel's, Brooks Bros.,* 492 A.2d 580 (D.C. App. 1985).

4. Annotation, Exchange Among Insurers of Medical Information Concerning Insured or Applicant for Insurance as Invasion of Privacy, 98 A.L.R.3d 561 (1993).

5. *See* Andrea Havens, "The Spleen That Fought Back," 20 *The Brief* 11, 40 (1990).

6. 51 Cal.3d 120, 271 CalRptr. 146, 793 P.2d 479 (Cal. 1990).

7. J. Bruce, *Privacy and Confidentiality of Health Care Information,* p. 56.

Appendixes

A

American Medical Association Confidentiality Statement

The information disclosed to a physician during the course of the relationship between physician and patient is confidential to the greatest possible degree. The patient should feel free to make a full disclosure of information to the physician in order that the physician may most effectively provide needed services. The patient should be able to make this disclosure with the knowledge that the physician will respect the confidential nature of the communication. The physician should not reveal confidential communications or information without the express consent of the patient, unless required to do so by law.

The obligation to safeguard patient confidences is subject to certain exceptions which are ethically and legally justified because of overriding social considerations. Where a patient threatens to inflict serious bodily harm to another person and there is a reasonable probability that the patient may carry out the threat, the physician should take reasonable precautions for the protection of the intended victim, including notification of law enforcement authorities. Also, communicable diseases, gunshot and knife wounds should be reported as required by applicable statutes or ordinances.

Section 5.05, *Current Opinions of the Council on Ethical and Judicial Affairs of the American Medical Association,* 1989. Reprinted with permission.

B

Text of the Proposed WEDI Health Information Confidentiality and Privacy Act of 1993

Title VI-Paperwork Reduction and Administrative Simplification Sec. 6001. Preemption of State Quill Pen Laws.

After 1994, no effect shall be given to any provision of State law that requires medical or health insurance records (including billing information) to be maintained in written, rather than electronic, form.

SEC. 6002. Confidentiality of Electronic Health Care Information.

(A) Promulgation of Requirements.

    (1) In general. The National Health Board shall promulgate, and may modify from time to time, requirements to facilitate and en-

sure the uniform, confidential treatment of individually identifiable health care information in electronic environments.

(2) Items to be included. The requirements under this subsection shall

    (a) provide for the preservation of confidentiality and privacy rights in electronic health care claims processing and payment;

    (b) apply to the collection, storage, handling, and transmission of individually identifiable health care data (including initial and subsequent disclosures) in electronic form by all accountable health plans, public and private third-party payers, providers of health care, and all other entities involved in the transactions;

    (c) not apply to public health reporting required under state or federal law;

    (d) delineate protocols for securing electronic storage, processing, and transmission of health care data;

    (e) specify fair information practices that assure a proper balance between required disclosures and use of data, including

        (i) creating a proper balance between what an individual is expected to divulge to a record-keeping organization and what the individual seeks in return,

        (ii) minimizing the extent to which information concerning an individual is itself a source of unfairness in any decision made on the basis of such information, and

        (iii) creating and defining obligations respecting the uses and disclosures that will be made of recorded information about an individual;

    (f) require publication of the existence of health care data banks;

    (g) establish appropriate protections for highly sensitive data (such as data concerning mental health, substance abuse, and communicable and genetic diseases);

    (h) encourage the use of alternative dispute resolution mechanisms (where appropriate); and

        (i)   provide for the deletion of information that is no longer needed to carry out the purpose for which it was collected.

    (3)   Consultation with working group. In promulgating and modifying requirements under this subsection, the board shall consult with a working group of knowledgeable individuals representing all interested parties (including third-party payers, providers, consumers, employers, information managers, and technical experts).

    (4)   Deadline. The board shall first promulgate requirements under this subsection by not later than six months after the date of the enactment of this act.

(B) Application of requirements.

    (1)   State enforcement of similar requirements. The requirements promulgated under subsection (a) shall not apply to health care information in a state if (a) the state has applied to the national health board for a determination that the state has in effect a law that provides for the application of requirements with respect to such information (and enforcement provisions with respect to such requirements) consistent with such requirements [(and with the enforcement provisions of subsection (c))], and (b) the board determines that the state has such a law in effect.

    (2)   Application to current information. The national health board shall specify the extent to which (and manner in which) the requirements promulgated under subsection (a) apply to information collected before the effective date of the requirements.

(C) Defense for proper disclosures. An entity that establishes that is has disclosed health care information in accordance with the requirements promulgated under subsection (a) has established a defense in an action brought for improper disclosure of such information.

(D) Penalties for violations. An entity that collects, stores, handles, transmits, or discloses health care information in violation of the requirements promulgated under subsection (a) is liable for civil damages, equitable remedies, and attorneys' fees (if appropriate), in accordance with regulations of the national health board.

Glossary

Accreditation. The act of approving an institution to operate as a healthcare provider.

Accreditation Manual for Hospitals. The Joint Commission on Accreditation of Healthcare Organizations' standards for accreditation of hospitals.

Accrediting organization. An entity, usually a governmental entity, that inspects healthcare facilities and grants them permission to operate.

Administrative agency. A governmental body other than a legislative or judicial body, such as the U.S. Department of Health and Human Services, that executes governmental policy in a particular area.

Administrative regulation. A rule issued by an administrative agency to regulate the area in which the agency was created to execute government policy. Courts rank regulations below statutes but still have the force of law.

Authentication. An attestation that something, such as a record, is genuine.

Consent. Voluntary agreement. Consent may be express (oral or written), or implied (demonstrated by silence or actions).

Credentialing. The act of approving a healthcare professional's access to healthcare facilities. The granting of hospital or other types of professional privileges.

False light. The tort of portraying another in an objectionable false image in the public eye.

Intrusion on seclusion. The tort of intruding or prying into another individual personal affairs.

Joint Commission on Accreditation of Healthcare Organizations. A private, nonprofit association whose purpose is to improve the quality of health care through a voluntary accreditation process.

Health Care Quality Improvement Act. The federal statute that establishes procedures for peer review, provides limited immunity for those who participate therein, and sets up a data bank to collect information on sub-standard practitioners.

Medical record. A record that identifies the patient and documents the care he or she received.

Medical staff. The group of physicians that the facility has authorized to practice in the facility and that enacts bylaws and medical staff rules governing the medical operations of the facility.

Medical staff privileges. The authorization to practice in a facility.

Minor. A person who has not yet reached the age of majority so as to be considered an adult by law.

Patient bill of rights. A government statute or regulation specifying rights of healthcare patients.

Peer review. Scrutiny of a healthcare professional by other such professionals to determine whether he or she is qualified to practice his or her profession in a facility.

Penumbra. A concept in constitutional law under which various rights are implied from the penumbra or emanations from the rights written into the constitution.

Peer review. The scrutiny of healthcare professionals by those with similar credentials to identify and remedy patterns of unacceptable patient care and/or to grant medical staff privileges to practitioners.

Physician-patient privilege. A law that prevents a physician (or other healthcare professional) from disclosing confidences of a patient without the patient's consent.

Privacy. The condition of being left alone or being secluded.

Privacy Act. The federal statute that limits governmental collection, maintenance, use, and dissemination of certain personal information.

Privacy, right to. The right to be left alone. It usually consists of three related rights: to be free from governmental or other interference, to be free from intrusion or observation into one's private affairs, and the right to maintain control over personal information.

Privileged communication or information. Information acquired by a physician or other professional in attending a patient that was necessary to treat the patient. Such information is inadmissible in evidence and may not be otherwise released without the patient's consent.

Public disclosure of private information. The tort of publicizing a matter concerning one's private life that would be highly offensive to a reasonable person and is not of legitimate concern to the public.

Quality assurance. The evaluation of the quality and appropriateness of patient care.

Record. As a noun, the preservation of information or data on some medium so that it may be read at some future time.

Regulation. A rule issued by a governmental agency other than the legislature. Unless a regulation conflicts with the constitution or a statute, it has the force of law.

Subpoena. A written command requiring a person to appear at a trial or other hearing and give testimony.

Subpoena *Duces Tecum*. A written command requiring the person to bring with him or her certain records or documents in his or her custody or possession.

Tort. A civil, as opposed to a criminal, wrong. One who commits a tort is liable to the victim for damages suffered thereby.

Utilization review. The act of determining whether medical care was appropriate or properly performed.

Bibliography

The American Medical Association. *A Compendium of State Peer Immunity Laws*, Chicago: AMA, 1988.

The American Medical Association. *HIV Blood Test Counseling: A.M.A. Physician Guidelines*, Chicago: AMA, 1988.

Annotation, Exchange Among Insurers of Medical Information Concerning Insured or Applicant for Insurance as Invasion of Privacy, 98 A.L.R.3d 561 (1993).

Jo Anne Czecowski Bruce, RRA. *Privacy and Confidentiality of Health Care Information*. Chicago: American Hospital Publishing, Inc., 1984.

B. Furrow, S. Johnson, T. Jost, and R. Schwartz. *Health Law: Cases Materials and Problems*, 2d ed. St. Paul, Minn.: West Publishing Co., 1991.

Andrea Havens. "The Spleen That Fought Back." 20 *The Brief* 11, 40 (1990).

Edna Huffman. *Medical Record Management*, 9th ed. Berwyn, Ill.: Physician's Record Co., 1990.

Joint Commission on Accreditation of Healthcare Organizations. *1994 Accreditation Manual for Hospitals*. Oak Brook Terrace, Ill.: JCAHO, 1994.

Philip Kurland. "The Private, I." *University of Chicago Magazine,* 7,8 (Autumn 1976).

Theodore LeBlang and W. Eugene Basanta. *The Law of Medical Practice in Illinois* (1986 and 1993 supplement). Rochester, N.Y.: The Lawyers Co-operative Publishing Co.

Christopher Morter. "The Health Care Quality Improvement Act of 1986: Will Physicians Find Peer Review More Inviting?" *Virginia Law Review* 74 (September 1988), p. 1115.

William Morton. "Are You Protected by the Peer Review Privilege?" *Legal Aspects of Medical Practice* 16, No. 8 (August 1988) pp. 1,8.

Robert S. Peck. *Extending the Constitutional Right to Privacy in the New Technological Age.* 12 *Hofstra Law Review* 893 (Summer 1984).

Jonathan Tomes. *Healthcare Records Management, Disclosure, and Retention: The Complete Legal Guide.* Chicago: Probus Publishing Co., 1993.

Jonathan Tomes. *Informed Consent: A Guide for the Healthcare Professional.* Chicago: Probus Publishing Co., 1993.

Jonathan Tomes. *Medical Staff Privileges and Peer Review: A Guide for Healthcare Professionals.* Chicago: Probus Publishing Co., 1994.

Samuel Warren and Louis Brandeis. *The Right to Privacy*, 4 *Harvard Law Review* 193 (1890).

Index

About the Author

Jonathan P. Tomes is a practicing attorney and author in Chicago. He has handled many criminal and civil cases, including medical malpractice cases. He also serves as an associate professor at IIT Chicago-Kent College of Law. Among the subjects he has taught is administrative law—the part of the law that deals with the rules and regulations that administrative agencies (such as the Environmental Protection Agency, Health and Human Services, the Occupational Safety and Health Administration, and so forth) issue to control publicly regulated businesses, such as healthcare providers and hospital law.

Before going to law school, Professor Tomes served as an infantry platoon leader in Vietnam, where he won the Silver Star and the Combat Infantry Badge, among other awards. Then he graduated first in his class at Oklahoma City University School of Law and won the Oklahoma Bar Association outstanding law student award. He is a member of the Illinois and Oklahoma bars. Following graduation, he served in the Judge Advocate General's Corps, U.S. Army, until he retired as a lieutenant colonel in 1988. While in the military, he served as prosecutor, defense counsel, and military judge before becoming chief of special claims, Tort Claims Division, U.S. Army Claims Service, where he was in charge of processing and adjudicating claims that occurred overseas against the military, primarily medical malpractice claims. That assignment led to his interest in healthcare law. The military rewarded his 20 years' service by awarding him the Legion of Merit, the second-highest service award in the military, upon his retirement.

Among Professor Tomes' publications are *Healthcare Records: A Practical Legal Guide* (HFMA, 1990), *Healthcare Records Manual* (Warren, Gorham & Lamont, 1992), *Understanding Healthcare Environmental Law* (HFMA, 1992), *Industry Regulation* (Probus/HFMA, 1993) *Informed Consent* (Probus/HFMA, 1993), *Healthcare Fraud, Waste, Abuse and Safe Harbors* (Probus/HFMA 1993), *Antitrust Law: A Guide for the Healthcare Professional* (HFMA, 1993), *Healthcare Records Management, Disclosure & Retention: The Complete Legal Guide* (Probus/HFMA, 1993) and *Medi-*

cal Staff Privileges and Peer Review (Probus/HFMA, 1994). He has also published articles in *Health Data Management, Healthcare Financial Management, Military Review, Boston University Annual Review of Banking Law, Richmond Law Review, Air Force Law Review* (the U.S. Supreme Court cited his article in this law review) and *The Practical Lawyer.*